The
Vitamin C
Connection

Also by Dr. Emanuel Cheraskin and Dr. W. Marshall
Ringsdorf, Jr., with Arline Brecher

Psychodietetics

The Vitamin C Connection

Dr. Emanuel Cheraskin
Dr. W. Marshall Ringsdorf, Jr.
Dr. Emily L. Sisley

1817

HARPER & ROW, PUBLISHERS, New York

Cambridge, Philadelphia, San Francisco,
London, Mexico City, São Paulo, Sydney

FIRST EDITION

Designer: C. Linda Dingler

Library of Congress Cataloging in Publication Data

Cheraskin, Emanuel, 1916–
    The vitamin C connection.

    Bibliography: p.
    Includes index.
    1. Vitamin C—Physiological effect.   2. Vitamin C—Therapeutic use.
I. Ringsdorf, W. Marshall.   II. Sisley, Emily L.   III. Title.
QP772.A8C48   1983   612'.399   82–48657
ISBN 0–06–038024–1

83 84 85 86 87 10 9 8 7 6 5 4 3 2 1

Contents

The
Vitamin C
Connection

Introduction

What this country needs is a good five-cent pill!—some "magic," easy-to-swallow little pellet that can slow aging, minimize heart disease, aid recovery from dozens of infectious and degenerative ailments, and inoculate us against countless health problems that stem from emotional stress and environmental pollutants.

THE GOOD NEWS

Happily, such a thing exists—in pill form, as supplemental powders, and, of course, in a number of foods. We'll discuss these foods, and what you can do to combat the bad effects of processing, transporting, packaging, and cooking. But for the most part much of what you will read in this book has to do with supplemental sources of the "magic" substance—usually as capsules or tablets.

We are speaking of vitamin C. Except when a differentiation is scientifically necessary, we will use the terms *ascorbic acid* and *ascorbate* interchangeably with *vitamin C*.

What Vitamin C Can Do

It does more than ward off the common cold. Vitamin C enhances many immune mechanisms and protects against the flu, bronchitis, respiratory problems, and other virus infections.

It safeguards hearts. Vitamin C plays a vital role in the entire heart and vascular system, including the arteries, veins, and

1

smaller capillaries. It combats capillary permeability and fragility; it inhibits the clumping of blood; it lowers fat and cholesterol levels; it improves circulation and reduces cardiovascular abnormalities.

It saves sight. Vitamin C lowers the risk of developing increased pressure within the eyeball (glaucoma), a principal cause of blindness.

It helps you keep your "bite." By inhibiting tartar formation, vitamin C prevents periodontal damage—that is, gum, socket, and jawbone problems that are far more serious than cavities.

It reverses some forms of infertility. As reported in several studies, childless couples became parents-to-be with the aid of ascorbic-acid supplementation.

It is a dieting aid. Vitamin C cuts the craving for sweets and helps control a wayward appetite.

It is a natural anesthetic. Vitamin C can kill many kinds of pain, including low-back pain. It decreases the severity of post-operative pain and shortens recovery time.

It promotes wound healing. Among its many biochemical reactions, vitamin C has been shown to promote the healing of wounds, ranging from small nicks to bad cuts.

It "does something" about the weather. The discomfort experienced by rapid fluctuations in temperature—as well as prolonged extremes of hot or cold—can be reduced by taking vitamin C. Vitamin C also relieves prickly heat and other rashes suffered during hot spells.

It is a natural laxative. Taken after meals, vitamin C ends constipation. It can also shrivel hemorrhoids.

It is a detoxifier. By ridding the body of accumulations of heavy metals (such as lead, cadmium, and nickel) and pollutants found in our air, food, and water, vitamin C acts as a useful environmental protector.

It helps people "come clean." Vitamin C is nature's "drug fighter." It helps people withdraw from various drugs—ranging from prescribed mood changers to addictive substances such as heroin. It does this by enhancing metabolism of the drug and muting both toxicity and side effects. It can also reverse bad side effects from drugs that are necessary to some individuals' existence (for example, L-dopa in people with Parkinson's disease).

It whips "fatigue." Sufferers of so-called iron-poor blood enjoy renewed energy when they fortify with vitamin C along with their iron supplement. It's also great for fighting jet lag.

It reduces insulin requirements in diabetics. In less severe cases, vitamin C may even enable diabetics to control their ailment by diet alone.

It counteracts food allergies. The antihistaminic action of vitamin C can enable people to tolerate foods they otherwise could not eat.

It cures certain skin diseases. Many industrial workers run the hazard of contracting various rashes and other skin disorders induced by toxic fumes or the handling of certain chemicals. Vitamin C's effectiveness against skin problems has been demonstrated.

It keeps you "young" for a longer time. With its antioxidant action at the cellular level, vitamin C slows the development of aging symptoms.

It protects against fractures and bone disease. Mostly because of its direct effect on collagen (we'll describe the process in this book), vitamin C has shown a remarkable capacity to help knit bone and to wage battle against such supposedly hopeless bone diseases as ankylosing spondylitis and osteogenesis imperfecta.

It aids recovery from serious kidney diseases, decreases the discomfort of arthritis, improves the quality of life in multiple sclerosis victims, and combats many other disorders. Going from more common ailments familiar to most people on to rather obscure genetic disorders, vitamin C has shown its powerful remedial or alleviating effects.

It inoculates against psychic stress. Anxiety drastically reduces the body's ascorbic-acid level. When good levels are restored, psychologic stability returns and one is protected against stress-related disorders.

It enhances sexual performance. By abetting the healthy functioning of the endocrine glands, vitamin C can improve your sex life.

It neutralizes some carcinogens. Cured meats and many other food products are preserved with some potentially dangerous additives. Vitamin C blocks the reaction between nitrites and proteins, so that the cancer-implicated nitrosamines are not formed.

It helps prevent and treat cancer. Some authorities believe that cancer is basically a collagen disease that develops as a secondary effect of a deficiency of ascorbic acid in tissue. Ascorbic acid is known to be essential to the body's manufacture of interferon, and has been demonstrated to retard the spread of cancer cells and to control cell division.

How Can It Do These Things?

Except for a few hints given above, we are leaving explanations and discussions for the rest of this book. You will read a lot about immune mechanisms, biochemical reactions, cell behavior, and other bodily processes that are directly and indirectly influenced by vitamin C. A few readers may find some of this information just a bit too scientific for their taste; they are free to skim such sections and concentrate on *what* C does rather than *how* it does it. But it's our feeling that the more educated people become about how their bodies work, the better off they'll be in judging the merits of various nostrums hawked to health-conscious consumers.

How Can One Be Sure?

We have taken great pains to document each statement made under the heading "What Vitamin C Can Do." And that's only the beginning. Many other health problems, diseases, disorders, wounds, and ailments are discussed.

The experimental and clinical data we describe are not the enthusiastic, wishful-thinking anecdotes of faddists. The studies we cite are serious, scientific investigations conducted by well-trained researchers and clinicians who have used methods and techniques calculated to yield findings that—of whatever nature!—are then reported in medical and other professional journals.

How Can Questions Be Answered?

We have also sought to provide rational answers to some questions about vitamin C you've always wanted to ask when there was no one around to answer. Samples are:

Can I take too much?
How do I know if I'm getting too little?
Can I be allergic to vitamin C?
What happens if I stop taking vitamin C?
Are there any circumstances when I *should* stop taking vitamin C?
Can I get by on C alone?

THE BAD NEWS

More often than not, all the good news about all the things that vitamin C can do gets drowned in a sea of confusion. The real truth gets held hostage while a philosophic tug-of-war rages between adherents of two extreme positions: those who claim vitamin C can do everything and those who claim it does nothing.

While this unfortunate slugging match takes place, a vast middle ground of solid scientific information is overlooked. So the average reader of newspaper and magazine accounts—no matter how health-conscious or consumer-oriented he or she might be—is simply unaware that a great mass of published scientific data substantiates C's unequaled role in helping people to get well or to stay well.

More bad news concerns the manner in which some authorities seem to exercise bias when they flex their muscles to do battle with C. In some quarters, positive findings about ascorbic acid are downgraded unless they stem from crossover, double-blind studies done over long-term periods and replicated in at least a dozen other research or clinical settings. (We'll explain these research-methodology terms later in the book.) On the other hand, purely anecdotal material written by doctors, or undergraduate laboratory experiments that "knock" vitamin C, are heralded as major breakthroughs—and they frequently are the subject of juicy reports in newspapers and other media.

What Can Be Done About This Situation?

You, yourself, can take an active part in clearing up the confusion about vitamin C. You can start by reading this book. In chapter after chapter you will find scientifically valid evidence that vitamin C does indeed act in all the ways we've just outlined—plus plenty more.

It's our firm belief that an educated public will provide a clear answer to health professionals who, for whatever reason, persist in maintaining that vitamin C is either valueless or of dubious worth. More scientific-minded readers may wish to consult some of the original reports we cite. In any event, documentation is here to tell everybody—health-care personnel and the public at large—what C can do, and how it does it. We also include descriptions of some studies that regard C in a less-than-enthusiastic way.

Vitamin C's connections to health and illness are myriad. We believe that, in organizing all the material as we've done here, this book will serve to clear up the confusion that's existed at least since Linus Pauling's book was released. We hope also that *The Vitamin C Connection* will open doors to even further research aimed toward showing how ascorbic acid can contribute to healthier living and longer lives.

1
Why C?

Positions. Lights. Action!

An anesthetized woman's vital signs are monitored as the surgeon's blade deftly cuts into the patient's distended abdomen.

Their eyebrows arching quizzically in marked contrast to the somber confines of surgical masks, operating-room personnel stare in wonderment.

There, right inside the woman's belly—surely the cameraman will use a zoom lens!—lies a large pool of unclotted blood.

An observer murmurs, "But the working diagnosis was endometriosis."

A young orderly asks, "What's endometriosis?"

The assistant explains, "Well, the lining of the uterus is called the endometrium. Sometimes a pathologic condition sets in and endometrial tissue grows outside the uterus—out in areas of the pelvic cavity."

This conversational aside for the benefit of the TV audience does not distract the surgical team. They had suspected an ovarian cyst. Now the pool of blood makes them think more in terms of what doctors like to call "heroic measures."

They decide to remove *both* ovaries, as well as the uterus and—for good measure—the appendix.

Fade to the next few months after discharge. The woman—let's call her Anne—continues to suffer terrific abdominal pain along with repeated bouts of abdominal bloating, belching, and indigestion.

Good scenario for a medically oriented soap opera? Perhaps. But the tragic fact is that this material did not come from a TV script. It comes from an actual case study that merited a full report in *The Journal of the American Medical Association.*

In August, four months after her first operation in April, Anne was readmitted. This time physicians theorized a bowel obstruction. During surgery, they located and straightened a small twist in the woman's lower intestine. Once again they encountered several areas within the pelvic cavity that were oozing blood. They cauterized visible "bleeders" and drained off accumulated blood.

But it didn't work. A year later, in September, our hapless patient returned—once again seeking relief from abdominal distention and cramping pains. When her abdominal wall was sliced, surgeons extracted 3000 ml of blood. That amounts to 3 liters: the better part of a gallon of liquid! In addition, her liver was blanketed with a series of blood- and fluid-filled cysts. Surgeons drained the cysts and hoped for the best.

If you can imagine the doctors' frustration, imagine Anne's— not to mention the increasing probability that her best friends were wondering if it was all "mental"!

In two short months, she showed up again with her familiar complaints: a swollen belly and chronic pains. After a diagnostic puncture revealed a new mass of fresh blood, the fluid was drained surgically.

Now, if this were a TV script, the Holiday Season would be marred by our unfortunate heroine's troubles and the continued concern of her loved ones, who huddle about a wilted and drooping tree that symbolizes the doctors' fears that this might be Anne's last Christmas. For it is only in January that the whole hospital routine resumes.

After drainage, tests showed countless blood tumors. Transfusions were ordered and Anne was transferred to a large university medical center. Here they found that the spleen was riddled with tiny blood cysts. They removed the organ.

Since no one had quite determined the *cause* of all this recurring bleeding, hematologists (blood specialists) were called in. When tests failed to uncover any abnormality, cancer was suspected. Fitting a TV scenario, it was thought to be a well-hidden, impossible-to-locate cancer.

In May, the symptoms returned. This time the pancreas fell under the dark veil of suspicion.

In yet one more year Anne came back again, presenting her by-now-long-term clinical picture. On June 12th, 4500 ml—that is, way over one gallon—of blood was drained from her abdomen. Biopsy showed widespread hemorrhaging, with many blood-filled cysts and a lot of clotting throughout the affected area.

The specialists ran out of answers. But, as Gertrude Stein might have put it: "What is the question?"

In March of the following year, a hospital physician thought to ask it: "What do you eat?"

Anne's answer solved the four-year-old medical mystery. Her diet was totally devoid of fresh fruits and vegetables. Ascorbic acid in her plasma? Near 0. All the operations, all the drainage, all the tests and other medical procedures had been unnecessary. Our long-suffering, diagnosis-eluding, real-life TV heroine was suffering from *scurvy*.

Anne was placed on a simple regimen of 1000 mg of vitamin C each day, and she returned to a normal, disease-free state—albeit missing some organs.

FROM SHIPBOARD TO BREAKFAST TABLE

How could Anne be subjected to so many medical blunders?

Scurvy was conquered such a long time ago modern doctors expect to confront it only in textbooks. There it's described as an ancient, dreaded, debilitating disease that occurs after prolonged vitamin C deficiency. The disease carries with it anemia, a marked kind of lethargic weakness, and spongelike gums. Worse, there's severe internal hemorrhaging that can be especially bad where fibrous tissues connect tendons and ligaments to bone joints.

In olden days it was a very common affliction among sailors who rounded a world just found to be round. Their diet was heavy on salted meat and next-to-nothing on fresh vegetables and fruits—especially citrus fruits. Many of the victims never made it beyond where the "flat" world had been thought to end. They were buried at sea. When Vasco da Gama passed the Cape of Good Hope in 1498, he had lost 100 of his crew of 160. In 1593, the English admiral Sir Richard Hawkins reported that scurvy took the lives of 10,000 men under his command.

In the middle to late 1700s seafarers learned the cure—and the prevention. They didn't know it was vitamin C—nor did physicians, until the substance was finally identified in 1911. But both groups accepted the seemingly strange idea that oranges, lemons, and limes (did you ever wonder about the origin of the slang word for British sailors, "limey"?) could rid whole populations from the curse of a long, painful death from scurvy.

So scurvy seemingly disappeared into the deep, dark past. And, although one might think that the highly-credentialed doctors who treated Anne ought to have recognized her problem for what it was, they did not.

This is not surprising. *Why* is it not surprising?

Many of today's doctors, much like their ancestral predecessors, are illiterate when it comes to nutrition. One survey showed that the average physician's secretary knows as much about healthy eating as her boss, except if she's on a diet. Then she knows *more!*

From their first days as medical students, doctors are usually not trained to regard malnutrition as a primary, or even contributing, cause of disease. Nutritional neglect is ignored as traditional medical-school curricula become increasingly geared toward specialization. Would-be physicians are taught to recognize one part of the body at a time, then one set of symptoms at a time, then one mode of therapy at a time. The *whole person* tends to get lost. Then, to top it off, complaints that "ought" to be recognized within the context of the whole person are frequently shunted off to the even more mysterious realm of what's considered to be psychosomatic ailments. Finally, traditional medical training relegates nutrition to about the same limbo as sunlight and fresh air, when it comes to factors directly related to health and illness.

Yet what of Anne herself? Was she blameless? Why would a middle-class, educated woman living in California—where citrus fruits and fresh vegetables are virtually in one's backyard year round—deliberately avoid eating all dependable sources of vitamin C?

In the final analysis, there is only one person responsible for your health and well-being: *you.*

A FRESH LOOK AT AN OLD CONCEPT

We'd like to see people assume more responsibility for their own bodies. It's hardly a new concept. It's redolent of wisdom preached by the ancients. Long before germs were dubbed the vexing villains that make us ill, when people got sick they assumed they had done something wrong. Health and disease were regarded as a sort of metaphysical justice meted out by the gods. When people behaved properly, they stayed well; when they broke rules, they were struck down.

As we'll detail in the last chapter of this book, vitamin C is not the sole answer to healthy living.

All the scientific knowledge painfully gained since the ancient behavior-illness connection does not negate the basic fact that each individual is substantially in command of his or her own medical fate. We know that health and disease result from an interplay between the environment and our own ability to cope with it. Whether people resist or fall to disease reflects in very large measure how carefully (or neglectfully) they have maintained their own bodies.

Many writers have addressed themselves to this "self-responsibility" theme, but none more eloquently than the late Dr. Jacques M. May. He wrote: "It is as though I had on a table three dolls, one of glass, another of celluloid, and a third of steel, and I choose to hit the three dolls with a hammer, using equal strength. The first doll would break, the second would scar, and the third would emit a pleasant sound."

Similarly, in an unfavorable environmental situation, the person who neglects his or her own physical condition will shatter like the glass doll. The individual who fortifies his constitution will, like the steel doll, shrug off the hammer blows of everyday stress and "sound good" doing so.

The Focus on Vitamin C

This principle of taking responsibility for fortifying one's body against the jolts of a threatening everyday environment has recently taken hold in the form of an American "fitness boom."

Many people have taken to running or jogging, biking or playing tennis, exercising (alone or in classes) or going to gyms. Some have given up cigarettes. Still others patronize health-food stores and gulp vitamins—taking extra C to ward off colds.

It's not a day too early! For all our emphasis on "health"—and our national pastime of keeping up with the latest advances in medicine, our world position is a national disgrace. A fifty-year-old American male has thirteen fewer years to live than a fifty-year-old man in Cyprus. When an American woman enters the labor room, she has less chance of surviving childbirth than her counterpart in eleven other countries. And her baby? The United States ranks a dismal fifteenth in infant mortality and nineteenth in male life expectancy at birth. All this is so despite the fact that we spend more money on medical research than all of the countries ahead of us.

This brings us back to self-responsibility. Somehow we're not doing enough. We need to do more, and we need to know more in order to do it.

This book focuses on vitamin C—also called ascorbic acid and ascorbate—for two very simple reasons.

1. Our lives depend on vitamin C. We can no more live without it than we can live without oxygen.
2. There are more than ten thousand published scientific papers that make it quite clear that there is not one body process (such as what goes on inside cells or tissues) and not one disease or syndrome (from the common cold to leprosy) that is not influenced—directly or indirectly—by vitamin C.

As outlined in our introduction and as detailed in the chapters that follow, vitamin C can inoculate a person against hundreds of environmental pollutants, infectious and degenerative diseases, and emotional distress that sometimes drives people into psychotherapy unnecessarily.

Sounds too good to be true?

In this book you'll find scientific evidence for all that vitamin C can do. This information has been obscured for too long a time by the scientific controversy that's been raging ever since 1970, when Dr. Linus Pauling said vitamin C is good for colds.

It is; but it is good for a lot of other things too.

The health-conscious reader who is willing to take some responsibility for his or her own health and well-being deserves a whole book that is focused entirely on vitamin C.

This is that book.

2
Vitamin C's "Vanishing Act"

If one were to lock up an airtight room and cut off all incoming air, every single inhabitant would be dead in a matter of some minutes. If one were to leave the air—along with other necessities—but deprive them of vitamin C, most of the people would be dead within a year.

Clearly, human beings are as dependent on vitamin C as they are on oxygen. Sure thing, the survival time is longer. But, as you will see in those chapters in which we discuss diseases that feature the vitamin C connection, the lingering death is likely to be marked by considerable pain and disablement.

Most animals have the capacity to manufacture this essential nutrient in their bodies. But people, members of the monkey-ape order, guinea pigs, and a very few other creatures do not. Scientists have proven that we don't have the enzyme, l-gulonolactone oxidase, that enables most animals to synthesize vitamin C automatically by a chemical transformation of sugar that occurs in the liver.

Whatever the precise chemical mechanism, it's certain that we cannot make our own vitamin C. Yet we cannot live without it. We must take it in.

The problem with this state of affairs is that—as bad luck would have it—vitamin C is quite unstable. Chemically fragile, it can be readily destroyed by oxidation. Oxidation is a common chemical process that involves the interaction of a substance with oxygen. What this *means* in terms of vitamin C is pretty much: "Now you see it, now you don't."

"Preserving the natural level of food nutrients" is what Profes-

sor R. F. Cain of Oregon State University calls one of "the principal responsibilities of the food scientist and food technologist."
One must consider the various phases of food acquisition, its processing, how it is stored, and how, ultimately, it is prepared for a
meal. Cooking can kill vitamins. So can exposure to light, air,
heat, and other environmental elements.

In a workshop concerned with food protection, Professor Cain
presented data that clearly show the unstability (U) and relative
stability (S) of various nutrients in neutral, acid, or alkaline foods
as well as effects of environment.

NUTRIENT	NEUTRAL (pH=7)	ACID (pH<7)	ALKALINE (pH>7)	OXYGEN OR AIR	LIGHT	HEAT	COOKING LOSSES RANGE (%)
Vitamin C	U	S	U	U	U	U	0–100
Thiamin	U	S	U	U	S	U	0– 80
Niacin	S	S	S	S	S	S	0– 75
Riboflavin	S	S	U	S	U	U	0– 75
Vitamin A	S	U	S	U	U	U	0– 40
Vitamin D	S	—	U	U	U	U	0– 30
Carotenes	S	U	S	U	U	U	0– 30

As you can see, vitamin C doesn't stand much of a chance—
unless certain precautions are taken or one takes supplements.

But, before we tackle the implications of vitamin C's vanishing
act, let's take a short quiz to see where we fit in the scheme of
things.

Tot up your YES answers. Although there is no precise point
value, it is safe to say that the more YES answers, the greater the
possibility that you have a special problem with vitamin C's vanishing act. The reasons will soon be evident. But first let's pause to
check some historical facts.

EARLY RUNS OF THE VANISHING ACT

As we noted in the previous chapter, citrus fruits' curative powers
were known to seafarers in the latter half of the eighteenth century.

Do you smoke?	YES	NO
Do you rarely eat fresh fruits and raw vegetables?	YES	NO
Are you taking a contraceptive pill?	YES	NO
Are you one who does not take vitamin supplements?	YES	NO
Do you take prescribed medications?	YES	NO
Do you rarely eat citrus fruit or juice?	YES	NO
Do you eat in restaurants frequently?	YES	NO
Do you dislike many of the green vegetables?	YES	NO
Are you under significant stress?	YES	NO
Are you bothered with chronic or recurring infections?	YES	NO
Do you bruise easily?	YES	NO
Have you been bothered with bleeding gums?	YES	NO
Are you required to take cortisone or other steroid drugs?	YES	NO

But so was their fragility. Way back in 1753 James Lind, the famous Scottish naval surgeon, pointed out that "as oranges and lemons are liable to spoil . . . the next thing to be proposed is the method of preserving their virtues entirely for years in a convenient and small bulk." E. J. Rolfe, of the National College of Food Technology at the University of Reading at Weybridge in Surrey (England), says that Lind "recommended the evaporation of the fruit juice in a clean open earthen vessel, well-glazed, for several hours on a water bath until the juice is a consistency of a syrup." Back to Lind himself: "It is then to be corked up in a bottle for use . . . so that thus the acid, and virtues of twelve dozen lemons and oranges may be put into a quart bottle, and preserved for several years." It worked.

THE VANISHING ACT'S CONTEMPORARY
PRODUCERS AND DIRECTORS

There is no question that Dr. Lind knew of C's vanishing act. But the show's run actually dates back to antiquity and beyond. Primitive people ate when they were hungry, assuming food was available. If it was, and the hunt had failed to produce an animal, eating consisted mainly of picking ripe fruit off a tree or mature vegetables from the earth. These goodies were consumed on the spot—no transporting, no processing, no enticing packaging, no fancy labels.

Today's scene is obviously more complex. Foods may be grown in special areas under exotic and often quite unnatural conditions. Pineapples won't grow on Martha's Vineyard, and people in New York City insist on Idaho potatoes!

Because of this geographic displacement and all the shipping involved, most of the popular foods on the market these days have undergone considerable—sometimes unrecognizable— change in the course of processing. Some essentials (and even what some people erroneously call *non*essentials) are removed. The fact that we "enrich" certain products is an admission that too much was taken out.

Let's watch Polly as she pushes her cart along the cavernous aisles of a large supermarket. She could just as well be Paul, and frequently is. But, since most family food shopping is still done by the woman of the household, let's stick with the female gender, with the understanding that Paul is no less subject to whim (or wisdom) than Polly.

The canned-food section is replete with approximately one dozen brands of tomatoes. One manufacturer has taken pains to replicate the most vivid hues of a Turner sunset. Which brand will Polly buy?

The boxed cereals, all "enriched," are lined up attractively. One manufacturer's label features two winsome, angelic children devouring the product with gusto. Which brand will Polly buy?

One could name hundreds of examples. Suffice it to say that Madison Avenue often spends a company's major advertising budget on food items that are the least nutritious.

HOW THE VANISHING ACT IS PERFORMED TODAY

The Where and How of Growing

Long before processing enters the picture, the nutritional value of foodstuffs is influenced by where and how the food is grown.

Robert S. Harris, former Professor of Biochemistry of Nutrition at the Massachusetts Institute of Technology in Cambridge, explains that if a nutrient or its precursor(s) are not in the soil, or are in short supply, they cannot show up in optimal concentrations in food that's grown in that soil. Dr. Harris concludes: the "nutrient content of freshly harvested edible plants varies. Usually this variation is less than severalfold, but on occasion it may exceed 20-fold."

The importance of soil quality can be appreciated when one becomes aware that foods grown in the United States do not always compare favorably with those grown in other countries—even those called "underdeveloped." For example, according to Harris, "a detailed examination of data on Mexican foods revealed that in a number of instances the variety of a food plant produced in Mexico was higher in nutritional value than the same food grown in the United States. The Latin American varieties were generally more nutritious.

"In his eagerness to produce more kernels per row, more rows per ear, and more ears per stalk, the plant breeder [in the United States] has sacrificed nutrient content. In his desire to produce lovelier apples, sweeter oranges, blander vegetables, shipment-resistant foods, he has often produced varieties which are less nutritious per pound."

But Dr. Harris adds the hopeful note: "It is usually possible to obtain all these desirable effects without impairing the nutritional quality, if the plant breeder adds the nutritional factor to his working equation." There's a definite vitamin C connection here because that nutrient is one of those that appear in Mexican foods in higher concentration than in American counterparts.

Ripening and Picking

The *when* also counts—that is, when is the food plucked from soil or tree? In other words, what does *ripening* have to do with the garden-to-gullet chain of events?

Many investigators have looked at this link. Studying tomatoes, an excellent source of vitamin C, two scientists at the Department of Food Science and Human Nutrition at Michigan State University in Lansing estimated that the 6.5 million tons of tomatoes produced annually in the United States could provide one-third of the present recommended dietary allowance (RDA) of vitamin C for all Americans. This is so because, on the average, each 100 grams of fresh tomato contains approximately 23 mg of ascorbic acid.

But, given current harvesting practices, the figures are of little more than academic interest. Why? These same researchers, Pantos and Markakis, point out that field-grown tomatoes reach their highest vitamin C content approximately six weeks after the flower opens and just before the fruit turns red. Yet tomatoes are customarily harvested at an earlier stage and shipped to market before they are ripe.

In a carefully plotted experiment, tomatoes were stored in temperature- and humidity-controlled stainless-steel cabinets. Pantos and Markakis report: "There is a decline in the ascorbic acid content of the tomatoes with time of storage at all temperatures . . . [those] left on the vine and analyzed when they were almost fully red . . . contained 24.8 and 25.2 mg per 100 grams of fruit. One week later, the fruit on the vine were overripe and contained 19.2 and 18.2 mg per 100 grams, respectively."

In short, plant-ripened fruit is best; overripe is bad; and artificial ripening is worst.

Potatoes? S. V. Bring and her co-workers at the Home Economics Research Department at the College of Agriculture of the University of Idaho sampled potatoes harvested in October and found a vitamin C value of about 30 mg per 100 grams. By February, the content had decreased to about 12 mg. So assuming the October-harvested potato will not reach your table until February, it will have lost about 60 percent of its vitamin C.

Species Difference An orange is not an orange is not an orange—no matter how sweet it smells. There may be a measurable difference in the vitamin C content of juice from navel and Valencia oranges grown in different sections of the country. And, according to Jorg Augustin at the University of Idaho, vitamin-C content in potatoes may range from 12 to 45 mg per 150 grams (wet basis). That means a difference almost fourfold, low to high.

Another hitch comes with the increasing mechanization of harvesting. People don't like to buy damaged fruits and vegetables. So growers have developed tomatoes with skins thick enough to resist machine wounds—but they have lower nutrient value.

Storage

In a book called *Vitamins: Their Role in Health and Disease*, J. Marks discusses how enzymes decompose vitamins in fruits and vegetables that are stored for periods of time. He says that vitamin C "is particularly liable to this type of destruction" and cites a one-third loss in apples stored only two to three months. There's an even greater loss in green vegetables. Marks's findings concerning the vitamin C content of potatoes are summarized below.

CONDITION	MG/100 G
Main crop freshly dug	30
Stored 1–3 months	20
Stored 4–5 months	15
Stored 6–7 months	10
Stored 8–9 months	8

John Krochta is a research agricultural engineer for the United States Department of Agriculture in Berkeley, California. Along with an associate, Bernard Feinberg, he reviewed various studies on nutrient losses in stored fruits and vegetables. When Candace Arthur interviewed Krochta for the publication *Nutrition Action*, she asked him what will happen to the vitamins in an apple that sits in a store or on a counter for a period of time. Krochta replied: "It depends on how it is handled, and what the variety of apple it is. I would say that apples and oranges left at room temperature for a couple of weeks would lose some of their nutrients, but not a whole lot. On the other hand, something leafy, like lettuce, would shrivel away to nothing. And that loss of moisture parallels loss of nutrients."

STORAGE TIME IN WEEKS (AT 3° C OR 36° F)	GOLDEN DELICIOUS APPLES (MG C/100 G APPLE)	BOSKOOP APPLES (MG C/100 G APPLES)
0	10	16
11	5	11
16	6	11
21	5	9
28	5	8

As the above material shows, an apple can easily lose as much as 50 percent of its vitamin C content. And, back to a leafy vegetable, Krochta contends that spinach will lose 29 percent of its vitamin C in only twenty-four hours when stored at 66° to 78° F. Even at lower temperatures (32° to 40°F), the loss will be 35 percent in one week. In fact, with freezing, spinach will be stripped of 63 percent of its vitamin C content.

Containers At the United States Citrus and Subtropical Products Laboratories in Winter Haven, Florida, John M. Sweet and colleagues found that juice stored in plasticized cardboard containers or waxed cardboard was at a decided disadvantage because "oxygen diffuses through the walls of these containers to hasten vitamin C breakdown."

The damaging influence of packaging on the nutrient value of foods could consume an entire chapter of a book. In fact, *Nutritional Evaluation of Food Processing* has just such a chapter. It's written by Marcus Karel, Ph.D., Professor of Food Engineering and Deputy Head of the Department of Nutrition and Food Science at the Massachusetts Institute of Technology in Cambridge, and Endel Karmas, Ph.D., Associate Professor of Food Science in the Department of Food Science at Rutgers University in New Brunswick, New Jersey.

At the risk of oversimplification, we'll attempt to summarize the situation. While glass containers continue to be used, both the availability of alternatives and the real need for certain qualities (for example, rigidity combined with pliability) combine to bring the world of technology into what holds our foods and liquids—plastics, silicone, plastic film, and metal foil, not to mention metals, paper, and wood.

The critical point is that packaging influences the nutritional content of foods. This involves factors such as light, oxygen concentration, moisture content, heat transfer, contamination, susceptibility to biologic agents and microorganisms, and even the interaction between package and food.

Heidelbaugh and Karen found many differences in how vitamin C content is affected by types of containers—tin, aluminum, and polyester film. Their findings are outlined in the two tables that follow.

Cranberry Sauce After Storage for Five Weeks at 37° C

	VITAMIN C (MG/100 G)
Prior to storage	89.20
No. 2 lined tin can	73.40
Aluminum laminate	71.72
Polyester film (2 layers)	0.40
Polyester film (1 layer)	0.00

Vegetables and Bacon After Storage for Five Weeks at 37° C

	VITAMIN C (MG/100 G)
Prior to processing	3.7
Prior to storage	3.0
Aluminum metal can	0.6
Aluminum laminate	0.6
Polyester film (2 layers)	0.0
Polyester film (1 layer)	0.0

Other Factors

Blanching As we've seen, even untreated (supposedly fresh) foods can lose nutrient value in storage. How about treated foods?

Sometimes the best of intentions go awry. Canned foods are routinely blanched—that is, exposed to boiling water or steam—to inactivate enzymes that might adversely affect the food. Unfortunately, total enzymatic inactivation is not normally possible with blanching—so the purpose may be at least partially defeated. (Blanching also removes gases and ensures vacuum conditions after filling and sealing.) Equally unfortunate for nutrition-minded consumers, blanching can cause a loss of vitamin C from 13 to 63 percent (depending on the length of exposure to high temperature).

Temperature An article in *Science News* described an experiment performed by the Winter Haven, Florida, research group mentioned previously. The researchers stocked shelves with single-strength canned grapefruit juice (that is, not the concentrate) and analyzed the effects of varying temperatures on juice stored for twelve weeks. While refrigerated juice lost little vitamin C value, that stored under hot warehouse conditions lost up to 70 percent of its potency.

Getting It There the Processed Way

Once all the various steps of growing, packaging, and storing are completed, we are faced with another problem. How does the food get to the supermarket and to you?

An unrivaled transportation network has made it possible to bring an almost inconceivable variety of foods to Americans throughout the year. So-called "fresh produce" must be shipped for long distances and stored for varying periods of time. In many major cities, it is quite rare nowadays to purchase locally grown food within twenty-four hours of its harvesting.

What this means, in essence, is that a very substantial portion of our population eats *processed foods.* How significantly does this influence our diet? Take the word of Professor Harris, an expert cited earlier. In the preface to the first edition of his book *Nutritional Evaluation of Food Processing,* Dr. Harris comments: "If food processing is defined to include all treatments of a foodstuff from the place of origin to the point of consumption, then more than 95% of our food is processed." He adds, "In most cases food processing causes a reduction of the nutritional value of a food."

Imagine: from the time food is plucked from the ground, a vine, or off a tree and the time we eat it, 95 percent has been processed in some way—all to our nutritional detriment. And, as if that were not bad enough, all the other factors we've discussed contribute to vitamin C's vanishing act.

Cooking and Serving

Once the food is grown and picked, stored in various containers, and subjected to other processing or packaging procedures before it is shipped long-distance by a vast transportation network, what then?

Well, back to Polly (or Paul). First of all, the food is bought. Scads of studies deal with what is purchased for household consumption—and, unfortunately, it seems that the intake of at least eight nutrients is only *two-thirds or less* than what the Committee on Dietary Allowances of the Food and Nutrition Board calls Recommended Dietary Allowances (RDAs)—amounts we believe (and this book will explain why) are too low to begin with. This appalling news comes from an investigation conducted by the late Agnes Fay Morgan, who was Professor Emeritus of Nutrition and Biochemistry at the California Agricultural Experiment Station at Berkeley.

Then, once the food is bought, it may be peeled, trimmed, and *over*cleaned until any nutritive value is run bone dry. And as for frozen foods, the necessary act of defrosting further robs them of nutrients.

But there's little doubt that the *most* harmful stage—and, interestingly, the one we are most able to control—occurs in cooking. Fortunately, quite apart from measures such as avoiding overcooking and/or eating more raw or undercooked foods, there's an easy way to get around this problem. Simply add crystalline vitamin C to your favorite recipes once they are prepared. It's quite easily obtainable at drug, health-food, and nutrition stores and can be sprinkled with impunity onto or into most anything you wish to serve.

Such an addition can be of crucial importance; the Department of Agriculture says cooking can account for as much as 50 to 55 percent of vitamin C loss. Then, to worsen things, the food tends to stand around after preparation—sometimes as long as hours. The results can be devastating. For example, when baked-in-the-skin potatoes sit at a steam table for thirty minutes, there is a 34 percent vitamin C loss. Within the next fifteen minutes, the loss rises to 59 percent. Potatoes that are peeled, cut in halves, steamed, and mashed or creamed show the following losses:

MINUTES AT STEAM TABLE	% LOSS
0	39
30	63
60	95

Mary K. Head of the Department of Food Science at North Carolina State University in Raleigh studied nutrient losses during preparation, distribution, and serving in school kitchens. She wanted to find out how much loss occurred during the foods' transfer in insulated carts, how much loss occurred in individual menu items before and after preparation, and how much loss occurred during the serving period. She noted that "major ascorbic acid losses were noted in most foods" with "the mean loss of 19% ascorbic acid from hot foods [causing] concern."

So evidence strongly suggests suboptimal C intake at school as well as in the home. But Americans also eat elsewhere, and the picture is about the same—as we'll see below.

Fast Foods Lest anyone doubt the importance of fast-food chains to the American diet, let him or her consider this true story told by Dr. Robert E. Klein, a dentist from Mansfield, Ohio.

Asked in a quiz to name the four basic food groups, a student answered: "McDonald's, Wendy's, Burger King, and Pizza Hut."

But the joke isn't so funny in terms of the economy. Estimates are that nearly 50,000 fast-food restaurants are selling food to the dining public, who on the average eat out between four and seven times a week. While the gourmand—let alone the gourmet— may wince, there are reasons for the increasing appeal of fast foods. The menu items are popular, filling, and inexpensive. The service is generally quick, the food is freshly prepared, and a level of quality can be maintained because of the limited menu. Customers can be reasonably sure the taste of the food won't vary from one location to another or from one day to the next because purchasing and preparation standards are highly controlled in the large chains.

Of course, as many publications (such as *Medical Times*) have pointed out, there are limitations in the nutritional value of fast foods. Along with a colleague, Ellen H. Brennan, and a consulting dietitian, Gaynell L. Irving, Eleanor A. Young, Associate Professor in the Division of Human Nutrition at the Department of Medicine in the University of Texas at San Antonio, set out to see just what this massive consumption of franchise food really means in terms of nutrition. The investigators concluded that "a typical meal provides approximately ⅓ of the RDA for thiamin, niacin, ascorbic acid, vitamin B_{12}, and vitamin D." (Again, as we emphasize throughout this book, there's a great deal of evidence to support our contention that C's 60-mg RDA is too low a figure.)

Here's a summary of the vitamin C content in McDonald's meals:

	MG VITAMIN C
¼-lb. hamburger, french fries, chocolate shake	20.0
Big Mac, french fries, chocolate shake	22.6
Cheeseburger, french fries, chocolate shake	21.3
Hamburger, french fries, chocolate shake	21.0

Since this table is representative of the ascorbic-acid level in foods supplied by the fast-food chains, we can see that, even in these high-calorie meals, vitamin C intake is only about one-third of the RDA.

Catering and the Hospital   Traditionally the catering industry drew most of its raw materials directly from the food producer, via the wholesale market. Now this generally occurs through the intermediary of the food manufacturer.

Ironically, one may have to be hospitalized to discover how bad catered food can taste. (We are not, of course, discussing the gourmet caterer who handles fancy social affairs.) But, aside from taste, nutritional value is often ruined by cooking practices. Investigators at the University of Leeds decided to investigate "the fate of frozen peas in a special diet kitchen in a 400-bed hospital for acute patients. Ninety-five per cent loss in ascorbic acid was observed." A table adapted from this report by Glew, Hill, and Millross summarizes the story.

Cooking Practice for Frozen Peas in a Hospital Diet Kitchen

TIME	PROCEDURE	ASCORBIC ACID MG/100 G
9:45 A.M.	Frozen peas sampled and put into boiling water	20.5
9:50 A.M.	Sample taken	15.0
10:20 A.M.	Water began to boil	
10:35 A.M.	Peas strained and put onto hot plate	8.1
11:10 A.M.	Sample from hot plate taken	3.7
12:10 P.M.	Sample taken at time of service to patients	1.1

Glew and co-workers observed similar practices and results in 152 other hospital kitchens surveyed. The larger the hospital, the longer the food preparation and serving time and the greater the loss of various nutritional elements such as vitamin C.

Among other studies are those by Richard A. Wright of the University of Louisville and the VA Medical Center there. Wright cites work by Bistrian and colleagues at the Boston City Hospital and by Willcutts at a private community hospital. In the former, more than 44 percent of the patients were malnourished; in the latter, 33 percent were malnourished. These disturbing rates seem almost good in comparison with Wright's own findings: "Our nutrition team found that more than 75 percent of the patients deviated from the norm by two or more anthropometric [size-weight-proportional measurements of a person] and laboratory determinations."

T. P. Eddy, investigating different-size and different-type hospitals, says that "defects in preparation and service damaged the food, causing nearly complete loss of vitamin C in potatoes and 75 percent loss in green vegetables." Eddy's findings are summed up in the table that follows.

Mean Values of Ascorbic Acid in Mg in the Three Main Meals Served in Various Sizes and Types of Hospitals

TYPE OF HOSPITAL	ACUTE			CHRONIC		MENTAL
Number of beds	1–100	101–300	>300	1–100	>100	
MEAL						
Breakfast	1.5	2.0	1.0	1.4	0.5	2.0
Lunch	29.0	15.0	12.0	10.0	9.0	16.0
Dinner	7.0	5.0	5.0	1.0	1.3	3.0

Way back in 1974, Time magazine (in its July 22 issue) published an article called "Deadly Hospital Food?" The piece quoted the nutritional expert Dr. Charles E. Butterworth, Jr., director of a major program at the University of Alabama in Birmingham and Chairman of the AMA's Council on Foods and Nutrition. "'I suspect,' writes Butterworth in *Nutrition Today*, 'that one of the largest pockets of unrecognized malnutrition in America exists not in the rural slums or urban ghettos, but in the private rooms and wards of our big city hospitals.'"

Dr. Butterworth's accusation comes from an intensive study of patients in an institution affiliated with the University of Alabama's Medical Center. Investigators found too much surgery being done without first building up the patients; doctors ignoring good nutrition and choosing the exclusive use of antibiotics to fight infection (a matter we'll discuss in the next chapter); and enough post-operation nutritional neglect for patients to become severely malnourished. The *Time* article continues: "Of 80 patients studied at the University of Alabama, 14 were hospitalized for more than 3 weeks without receiving vitamin supplements, although their symptoms suggested that they might have been undernourished."

Unfortunately, the situation hasn't changed much over the years and this is downright ominous when one considers that—based on government figures released in 1979—about 22 million Americans per year spend around ten days in a hospital.

The Upshot of It All

Vitamin C's vanishing act has perhaps been best described by Dr. Robert S. Harris. He says that "by the time that processed foods reach you, they may have been shipped and stored, trimmed, blanched, frozen, canned, condensed, dehydrated, pasteurized, sterilized, smoked, cured, milled, roasted, cooked, toasted or puffed. What's left of their composition after any combination of those tortures is then liable to be further stolen by heat, light, oxygen, oxalates, antivitamins, acidity, alkalinity, metal catalysts, enzymes, and irradiation."

THE INTERNAL PROBLEM

As hazardous as all these external problems are, the problem is *not all out there!* Vitamin C can vanish during absorption, assimilation, and utilization by the body. Here are some things that contribute to the "internal" vanishing act.

Contributing Factors

Smoking With the possible exception of major cigarette manufacturers, few people would deny the magnitude of the health hazard posed by smoking. As most people know, the real popularity of cigarettes (as opposed to cigars, pipes, chewing tobacco, and snuff) is a post–World War I phenomenon. Recent figures translate into over 4000 cigarettes each year—more than half a pack per day—for every American over the age of eighteen. W. J. McCormick calculates that one cigarette "burns up" 25 mg of vitamin C. This means someone smoking half a pack of cigarettes a day is destroying 250 mg of vitamin C.

What if you don't smoke? James R. White and Herman F. Froeb of the University of California at San Diego say that nonsmokers can be sharing someone else's cigarette whether they like it or not. "And the smoke does more than get in your eyes," they wryly add. White and Froeb describe a *Lancet* report. The study compared the nicotine content in the urine of smokers and of nonsmokers placed in an unventilated room filled with cigarette smoke. In the latter group, the nicotine concentration was almost 80 percent of the lowest figure in the range found for smokers. That's just about like smoking!

United States Government publications ignore smoking's vitamin C connection. Yet a summary of the scientific literature on this subject was published years ago by a scientist, Omer Pelletier, at the Nutrition Research Division of the Food and Drug Directorate in Ottawa. Pelletier confirms the connection and suggests that "smokers would need about twice as much vitamin C as nonsmokers to maintain comparable [blood] levels."

Even earlier, we had undertaken to study the smoking–vitamin C connection not only by measuring blood plasma levels but also using an intradermal injection test in volunteer dental students. In this latter technique, we introduced a small amount of harmless blue dye into the skin and noted the minutes required for the blue discoloration to disappear. The faster the disappearance of the dye, the greater the amount of vitamin C in the skin. We measured two things: (1) the plasma level of vitamin C at various times and (2) the time it took for C to counteract the dye's effect.

Plasma Vitamin C Levels (mg%) Before and After IV Injection of 1 g Vitamin C

	NONSMOKERS	SMOKERS
Initial	0.72	0.39
After injection:		
15 seconds	1.25	1.26
24 hours	1.16	0.89
48 hours	1.15	0.80

The findings are clear: smoking adversely affects the absorption and utilization of vitamin C. But a few points bear special mention. First, as Dr. Pelletier had assumed, the initial vitamin C blood level of nonsmokers is approximately twice that of smokers.

Blue-Dye Disappearance Time (Minutes)
Before and After IV Injection of
1 g Vitamin C

	NONSMOKERS	SMOKERS
Initial	20.1	26.1
After injection:		
15 minutes	9.8	12.3
24 hours	19.1	21.1
48 hours	18.7	26.3

In both groups, it rises after the intravenous injection of 1 gram of C (about equivalent to the C content in approximately twelve glasses of orange juice). But the higher levels are *maintained* in nonsmokers.

Apart from risking other health hazards, the smoker brings an internal factor that adds to a loss of vitamin C—much of which has already vanished because of garden-to-gullet deterioration.

"The Pill" and Other Pills Despite the clearcut advantages of oral contraceptives, an unnatural body condition is induced. The human organism was not designed to live in what the Population Information Program at Johns Hopkins dubbed "a state of perpetual pregnancy." That, from a metabolic standpoint, is essentially the situation faced by the oral-contraceptive user.

A few researchers—including M. K. Horwitt and colleagues at St. Louis University in Missouri and the team headed by Ananda S. Prasad at Wayne State University in Detroit—believe that vitamin C metabolism is either minimally or not at all influenced by "the pill."

But the overwhelming consensus is that there is a definite connection. From the Department of Human Nutrition and Food of the New York State College of Human Ecology at Cornell University in Ithaca, Jerry Rivers—working alone and with Marjorie M. Devine—noted decreased ascorbic-acid concentrations in oral-contraceptive users as compared with controls. Reduced levels were also noted by Victor Wynn of the Alexander Simpson Laboratory for Metabolic Research at Saint Mary's Hospital Medical School in London. Wynn says that women using "the pill" "would have to take about 500 mg of vitamin C daily to normal-ize blood and tissue levels."

As to increasing reports of adverse side effects and the contro-versy about risk-benefit ratio, we quote two researchers whose report was published in the distinguished scientific journal *Na-ture*. Michael and Maxine Briggs maintain: "It is possible that some of the reported side-effects of 'the pill' may be a conse-quence of this vitamin lack."

Perhaps women who opt to continue taking an oral-contracep-tive pill may want to counteract this loss by taking a vitamin C supplement.

But how about other pills? According to data from the National Health Survey (Series 10, Number 131) "Aspirin or aspirin-type pills were estimated to have been used by 94 million persons 20 years of age and over during the 6 months preceding the inter-view."

Various researchers have agreed that aspirin has a bad effect on vitamin C metabolism. As long ago as 1936, Amy L. Daniels and Gladys J. Everson, from the Department of Nutrition, Iowa Child Welfare Research Station, at the State University of Iowa, discov-ered that aspirin increases the urinary excretion of vitamin C in children—that is, it depletes the body's store. This storage drain was confirmed at the New York University College of Medicine by J. M. Spitzer and Shepard Shapiro, who worked with children and adults, and by M. A. Sahud and R. J. Cohen at the University of California in San Francisco, who worked with forty-eight nor-mal subjects and thirty-four arthritic patients. The latter study showed that both plasma and platelet vitamin C contents were harmed by aspirin but that when arthritics on high aspirin doses also took vitamin C on a daily basis levels were comparable to those in normal subjects.

Another study is of special interest because it dealt with healthy students who volunteered to take doses of aspirin ranging from those generally used for simple headache or fever up to those taken in an attempt to relieve extended chronic pain. Even a sin-gle dose of aspirin inhibited uptake of vitamin C by white blood cells. (This is important to infection and disease, as we'll describe in the next chapter.) It also caused urinary excretion of vitamin

C. The larger the dose, the worse the effects. In fact, the researchers—a group from the Department of Pharmacology at Ireland's University of Dublin, headed by H. S. Loh—found that not even 500 mg of vitamin C added to 600 mg of aspirin was enough to enhance the ability of white blood cells to accept C. They recommended several daily C supplements be given to persons who take aspirin for several days at a time or longer.

To date, not much work has been done on the bigger problem of drugs in general. We expect further C connections to emerge when the same time, energy, and money are spent studying non-aspirin compounds as has been spent on investigating aspirin. In any event, there is no evidence to indicate that there is *not* such a connection (read our information on antibiotics in the next chapter, for example). So we have every reason to believe that the vitamin-C connection applies to *all* drugs—medicinal and otherwise—and we urge readers to consider how they, themselves, might unwittingly be contributing to vitamin C's vanishing act.

As to whether such a thing—the vitamin C vanishing act—exists, we rest our case. But supplementation can conquer this problem for those who can't grow their own food. And for people who, for whatever reason, dislike taking pills or tablets in general, sprinkling crystalline vitamin C onto food is an excellent way to return the vanished C.

3

How Not to Be
Bugged by Infections

Counting all the microorganisms that can cause infection is a little like trying to guess how many pebbles are in a giant container—and then discovering the container has no bottom.

It's easier to count the number of people who are bugged by these nasty body invaders. In one recent year, for every 100 inhabitants of the United States, there were 45.9 common colds and 42.9 influenza-like ailments. Other infectious diseases struck 24.2 times for every 100 persons.

How about the Americans who escaped the bugs? As you may have gathered by now, there's a definite vitamin C connection. But more of that later. First, let's check how prone *you* may be to infection. See the quiz on the next page.

The more YES answers you circled, the more likely you are to be infection-prone.

Later in this chapter we'll discuss several infectious diseases—except for the common cold, which you can read about in Chapter 7. Meanwhile, let's probe some of the body's coping mechanisms and some research findings that explain some of vitamin C's connections.

THE BODY'S COPING MECHANISMS

Immunity

Antibodies are blood-carried protein substances said to be "antagonistic" to infectious organisms like bacteria and viruses. They

Do you have at least one cold each year?	YES	NO
Does a cold occasionally worsen and require medical attention?	YES	NO
Do small cuts and scrapes frequently become infected?	YES	NO
Have you a family history of diabetes?	YES	NO
Do you have diabetes?	YES	NO
Would you say that the time required for you to heal is greater than average?	YES	NO
Do you occasionally have an infection of the gums around the teeth?	YES	NO
Have you had pyorrhea?	YES	NO
Have you had the flu more than once?	YES	NO
Have you ever had pneumonia?	YES	NO
Have you ever had skin boils that require a doctor's attention?	YES	NO
Are you allergic to one or more antibiotics?	YES	NO
Do you have other allergies?	YES	NO
Have you had infections that resisted antibiotic treatment?	YES	NO
Do you have a condition that necessitates your receiving an antibiotic regularly or periodically?	YES	NO
Have your tonsils been removed?	YES	NO
Have you had chemotherapy for cancer?	YES	NO
Do you avoid citrus fruits or juices?	YES	NO
Do you consume sweets (soft drinks, candy, desserts) several times daily?	YES	NO
Do you abstain from taking vitamins?	YES	NO

Women should also answer these two questions:

Are you bothered with a recurring urinary bladder infection?	YES	NO
Do you periodically have a resistant or recurring vaginal infection?	YES	NO

do more than "antagonize" these foreign substances—they help to
inactivate or kill them. Varieties you are most apt to read or hear
about being enhanced by vitamin C are immunoglobulin A (IgA);
immunoglobulin G (IgG); and immunoglobulin M (IgM). These
and other antibodies are produced by white blood cells called B-
lymphocytes.

There are other artillery batteries along the line of defense that
are beefed up by vitamin C. Prostaglandin E_1 (PGE_1) is a hor-
mone-like substance that's formed in human blood platelets. It
boosts T-lymphocytes, infection fighters produced in the thymus
gland. A blood chemical called C-3 complement seems to help
trigger B-lymphocytes to manufacture more antibodies and it also
mobilizes neutrophils (the most common white blood cell) and
helps these cells kill microbes. Leukocytes (lymphocytes and neutrophils) wander about the body, reconnoitering for bad-guy invaders. Interferon, a body chemical that interferes with viral proliferation, is also increased by vitamin C.

The nuts and bolts of immunology are, of course, far beyond
the scope of this chapter. Indeed, they can form (and have
formed) whole textbooks. But this brief introduction to immune
mechanisms should suffice here—except to say that experts frequently speak of two types of immunity. *Humoral immunity*, as
you might guess, involves antibodies that travel about through the
circulatory system. *Cell-mediated immunity* occurs when a particular cell destroys a microorganism or an abnormal cell.

Antihistamine Activity

Histamine is a body chemical that's released in response to any
kind of stress—physical, infectious, and otherwise. This increase
in circulating histamine can set off many reactions: heightened
secretion of stomach acid, a faster heartbeat, a drop in blood pressure, and constriction of breathing.

In respiratory infections, for example, histamine may dilate the
blood vessels. This causes them to leak fluid, which results in
swelling of the mucous membranes. Your nose runs; engorged tissues fill up your nose, making it difficult to breathe. Sinus membranes swell and sinus cavities are flooded with fluid. Your eyes

itch and water. Breathing can be further impaired if histamine causes enough muscle constriction to reduce the diameter of the bronchial tubes, air passageways to the lungs.

What's needed? Something to fight against the noxious chemical: an *antihistamine*. One guess: What has been shown to be an effective antihistamine? Right! Vitamin C. A chemical structure in histamine may be likened to a five-sided building. Ascorbic acid breaks through the walls, so the building is no longer functional. Antihistamine drugs work differently; they cling to cell membranes, offering protection from the histamine.

The rub is that the stress that produces the histamines also lowers vitamin C levels in the body. Since human beings cannot synthesize ascorbic acid, a natural means of combating histamine and its effects is lost. Later, we'll discuss how vitamin C supplementation can fight histamine directly and also make other antihistamines more effective.

Beefing Up Antibiotics

We've already outlined how the body's own coping mechanisms fight harmful microorganisms. There is also evidence that ascorbic acid has its own growth-inhibiting effect against these bugs. Additionally, it stimulates production of other, natural antibacterial factors and potentiates antibiotic medications.

When "outside" antibiotics are taken, two interesting things occur. The body's vitamin C is depleted (so that more is needed). And, when more is taken, it enhances the antibiotic's activity.

How this occurs, and how—in general—vitamin C prevents infections from bugging you will be explained below as we outline findings of some important research studies.

RESEARCH FINDINGS

Some General Connections

Because it activates body defense mechanisms mentioned above, vitamin C is effective against many viruses. From an extensive review of medical and scientific literature, Dr. Linus Pauling concludes that vitamin C combats a number of viral disorders: hepatitis, measles, mumps, poliomyelitis, viral pneumonia, viral orchitis (an inflammation of the testes), herpes zoster (shingles), herpes labialis (fever blisters), certain types of meningitis, influenza, and the common cold. The vitamin seems to exert both a preventive and a therapeutic effect when it is taken in the proper amounts, as we'll discuss in various sections of this book.

What about bacteria that seem to stalk an unprepared public? In his book *The Healing Factor: Vitamin C Against Disease*, Irwin Stone describes the role of ascorbic acid in bacterial infections; we summarize below.

VITAMIN C DOES THIS	WHICH MEANS THAT
It is bactericidal or bacteriostatic	It kills the baddies. It stops them in their tracks.
It detoxifies bacterial toxins	It "de-poisons" them, or renders them harmless.
It controls/maintains phagocytosis	It enables those cells that engulf and devour bacteria to enjoy the kind of dinner they like best.

According to research reports, vitamin C works against the bacteria and toxins of tuberculosis, diphtheria, tetanus, staphylococcal infections, dysentery, typhoid fever, leprosy, and pseudomonas infection.

The attack plan is similar for both antiviral and antibacterial campaigns. Ascorbate and molecular oxygen form a free radical (of the chemical variety!) in reactions that are catalyzed (facilitated) by copper ions present in the body. These radicals then launch a counter-offensive to immobilize or kill the invaders.

The Immunity Connection

Vitamin C has a powerful influence on the defense mechanisms of the body. With an eye to licking more than one kind of cold, S. Vallance spent a year on a British base in Antarctica. He gave his subjects 1 gram of supplementary ascorbic acid every day and noted a statistically significant increase in IgG and IgM.

A group of scientists from the University of Witwatersrand Medical School (Johannesburg, South Africa) gave 1 gram of ascorbic acid per day to twenty-five healthy male university students over a period of seventy-five days. Their findings, reported with Prinz as the first author, confirm several things. Vitamin C is vital for the two antibodies IgA and IgM, and also for the infection-fighting chemical C-3. The control-group students *not* given the vitamin showed no change in the blood-serum levels of IgA, IgM, or C-3.

Investigating cell-mediated immunity, Goetzl and co-workers incubated ascorbic acid with human neutrophils. The vitamin increased these cells' capacity for movement and their chemical attraction toward microorganisms (chemotaxis) by a whopping 100 to 300 percent. Vitamin C's enhancement of the ability of neutrophils to search and find inflammatory stimuli was also reported by an Indiana University School of Medicine (Indianapolis) team headed by Boxer.

This was confirmed in five healthy adult volunteers by Anderson and his associates at the Institute of Pathology at the University of Pretoria (South Africa) by giving the subjects 1 gram of ascorbate each day of the first week, 2 grams daily the second week, and 3 grams on every day of the third week. They found that after the people took 2 or 3 grams of vitamin C, neutrophils swung quickly into action against a bacterial toxin. No change was observed at the lower dose.

This same research group also experimented with 1, 2, and 3 grams of daily ascorbate to see whether more lymphocytes would be produced by the blood chemical mitogens (agents that enhance cell division), phytohemagglutinin, and concanavalin A. The answer: yes.

In still another study, Anderson and his colleagues worked with ten asthmatic children. A daily gram of ascorbic acid had two positive results. It brought neutrophil activity back to normal vigor. It also restored lymphocyte production to a normal rate.

Lymphocytes search and destroy invading bacteria and malignant cells. The mechanisms of lymphocyte production are complicated. But they interest experts who need to understand how ascorbic acid contributes to a process called *phytohemagglutinin-induced blastogenesis*, or, in plain English, cell division that re-sults in a rapid increase of lymphocytes.

The first group to report on this subject was Yonemoto, Chre-tien, and Fehniger from the National Cancer Institute and the City of Hope Medical Center in Duarte, California. They found that five healthy human subjects who took 5 grams of vitamin C each day for three days had a *twofold* increase in the rate of lymphocyte production. These findings were confirmed by Panush and Delafuente in a study of eighteen healthy subjects divided into three groups given the following: 1 daily gram of ascorbic acid; 3 daily grams; and a placebo (dummy pill) each day. Both vitamin C groups "won."

This mechanism may also explain how the body recovers from viral infections. Two researchers from Rochester School of Medi-cine, John P. Manzella and Norbert J. Roberts, Jr., took lympho-cytes and monocytes (two types of white blood cells) from healthy young adults and incubated them with phytohemagglutinin, the blood chemical that stimulates division of white blood cells (leu-kocytes). This cell division and circulation of leukocytes is known to be aided by vitamin C. But the action is depressed by the influenza virus. So some of the cells were infected with influenza virus. Then samples were treated with ascorbic acid equivalent to blood levels in people taking multigram doses. The researchers found that vitamin C blocks the influenza-induced reaction.

Other evidence continues to highlight vitamin C's starring role in immunity. At George Washington University School of Medi-cine, biochemists Gary B. Thurman and Allan Goldstein found that the vitamin can set off immune responses in infected ani-mals. In guinea-pig experiments, both the humoral and cell-medi-ated defense mechanisms were depressed in C-deficient animals. Those animals that survived required at least a month to recover after vitamin C was restored to their diet. These same research-ers, translating guinea-pig findings to the human realm, believe that ten to twenty times the supposed RDA (60 mg) for vitamin C is needed to ensure that a person has full immune competence.

Other lines of defense involve interferon—a body chemical

that interferes with the spread of viruses. Two Norwegian scientists, Helen Dahl and Miklos Degre at the University of Oslo, say interferon increases as vitamin C increases. This echoes findings of Benjamin Siegel (University of Oregon Health Sciences Center in Portland), who worked with cells from lower animals. He maintains that interferon does not work directly against viral invaders. Instead, it is produced by the cell under attack and then disperses out to surrounding cells. Those cells, in turn, produce another substance that prevents viral reproduction. The significance of interferon, according to Dr. Siegel, is that it works against *all* viruses and there's more of it when there's more vitamin C.

Carlton and Patricia Schwerdt at Stanford University incubated cultures of human cells with vitamin C for two days and then added the common cold virus (rhinovirus). The vitamin concentration equaled that in a person who is taking 6 to 10 grams of C daily—an amount that, no surprise to us, did not in any way hurt the cells. According to the Schwerdts, the rhinovirus went through one cycle of growth, and then was inhibited—probably as an effect of interferon. Forty-eight hours after the infection procedure, the amount of virus collected from the vitamin C culture was only one-fortieth the size of that from untreated control cells.

Another infection-preventing substance, known as NLAF (nonlysozyme antibacterial factor), is in normal tears. So is ascorbic acid. Several years ago Jack M. Holder designed a study to find out whether there was any relationship between the two substances.

The seventeen participants ranged in age from fifty-three to seventy-eight. Nonstimulated tears were collected with cellulose sponges and transferred to filter-paper disks. The disks were then placed on agar plates coated with a culture of *Micrococcus lysodeikticus*. These plates were incubated for forty-eight hours at 37° C before they were examined. The objective was to see how much the growth of the organisms had been inhibited in three sets of subjects. The method was measuring the diameter of the area. A zone measuring 22.5 mm would be considered normal.

SUBJECTS	DIAMETER RANGE	DIAMETER MEAN
8 patients with blepharitis (inflamed eyelids)	12.0–20.5 mm	17.6 mm
5 "normals"	20.0–25.0 mm	23.0 mm
4 subjects taking at least 250 mg of ascorbic acid daily	26.5–35.0 mm	30.6 mm

In the last group, the increase in size of inhibition zone was directly proportional to the amount of ascorbic acid taken—that is, the more the better from 250, through 300, through 500, to 1000 mg for the high point of 35.0 mm. The largest zone among the blepharitis patients (20.5 mm) was found in tear material from the one patient who was taking a modest dose—50 mg daily—of vitamin C.

These results suggest that ascorbic acid stimulates production of the antibacterial factor in tears. The implication for those thousands of people who suffer from eye infections is obvious.

The Antihistamine Connection

Histamine can restrict air flow. In a study in which each subject served as his own control, changes in airway caliber were assessed before and after histamine inhalation. On "the ascorbic acid day," each participant took an oral solution of 500 mg of vitamin C. The histamine inhalation and breathing-function measurements were repeated three and six hours later. After four or five days, the same basic procedure was followed—but a placebo (fake) was used instead of ascorbic acid. Zuskin and her colleagues at the Yale University Lung Research Center report that the vitamin C definitely inhibited the histamine effects (that is, the constriction of airways). This relief lasted about six hours.

Valic and Zuskin achieved similar results with people exposed to textile dusts and patients with symptoms of byssinosis (a syndrome caused by inhaling textile dusts). Since these dusts contain a material that releases histamine, the ascorbic acid may work against histamine's effect on smooth muscle. But vitamin C may also involve other mechanisms such as decreasing the permeability of tiny blood vessels. This would decrease the accumulation of fluid and any narrowing this may cause in the bronchial tubes.

The Antibiotic Connection

In addition to stimulating the body's defense mechanisms, vitamin C can fight microorganisms by cooperating with antibiotic medications. Rawal and his co-workers at the University of Queensland in Australia demonstrated that ascorbic acid, acting on its own, can inhibit the growth of sixteen strains of a particularly dangerous organism called *Pseudomonas aeruginosa*. But they also showed that the vitamin perks up the action of several prominent antibiotics: trimethoprim, sulfamethoxazole, ampicillin, erythromycin, polymyxin E, chloramphenicol, and the combination of trimethoprim and sulfamethoxazole (Bactrim or Septra). Perhaps of even greater interest: Septra, Bactrim, ampicillin, and erythromycin have no effect of their own against *Pseudomonas aeruginosa*. But, when they are accompanied by vitamin C, they show a statistically significant killing power.

These same Australian researchers applied their findings to six subjects with cystic fibrosis. When antimicrobials were administered along with vitamin C, the numbers of live microbes were reduced tenfold to one-hundredfold.

Surely the reader does not need us to underscore the fact that the antibiotics alone did not kill this microorganism. Since there is good evidence *for* taking vitamin C whenever antimicrobials are needed—and none against the practice!—it makes sense to play it safe.

The Connection to Some Specific Diseases

Allergies and Abruptio Placentae   Skin reactions of an allergic nature are usually initiated by a sudden release of histamine. Three Dublin-based researchers—Wilson, Loh, and Watters of the Department of Pharmacology at Trinity College and the Allergy Immunology Clinic at Mercers Hospital—believe that vitamin C uptake by leukocytes is a sensitive indicator that an allergic reaction results from histamine release. Leukocyte uptake suggests the need for supplemental vitamin C—which is what James A. Jackson at Sydenham Hospital in New York City prescribed for 68 rash-affected patients being prepared for oral surgery. These individuals happened to be suffering from itchy rashes (allergic reactions) about the mouth and face. Under a regimen of 250 mg of ascorbic acid twice daily for seven days, the itchiness and rashes subsided—but the reactions reappeared after the seven days, when the patients again confronted the allergens.

Though not an "allergic reaction," abruptio placentae is mentioned here because of its relationship to histamine. Histamine can induce muscle spasms of the uterus, rupturing the life-supporting membrane that surrounds a fetus. Alan Clemetson of Methodist Hospital in Brooklyn, New York, reports that expectant mothers can protect themselves and their unborn babies from abruptio placentae by taking daily doses of vitamin C.

Asthma   At the Yale University Lung Research Center, Kreisman, Mitchell, and Bouhuys evaluated the effects of inhaled histamine in seven subjects with bronchial asthma. Each participant received 500 mg of ascorbic acid four times daily for three days before "the histamine challenge." Results failed to measure up to ascorbic acid's reputation for counteracting histamine's constricting effects. But in the same lab it had been shown that this action lasts only about six hours, as we noted earlier. In this experiment the ascorbic-acid intake was withheld for twelve hours before the histamine inhalation. Kreisman and co-workers comment: "The protective action of ascorbic acid may be temporary, occurring shortly after single high doses (as in the previous studies)."

Another group of asthmatic patients was studied by a research team from the Department of Medicine at Johns Hopkins University—Kordansky, Rosenthal, and Norman. Three patients received 250 mg of ascorbic acid twice a day for a period of a week, and then an equal dose of a dummy substance for a week. Another three patients received the placebo first and then the ascorbic acid. On "ragweed challenge day," each person was given the ascorbic acid or the placebo three hours before the challenge. The experimenters reported that vitamin C had no protective effect. But we feel this study suffers from the same flaw in experimental design as the one described just above. Namely, the small dosage of vitamin C administered three hours before the ragweed antigen was simply not sufficient to maintain good tissue levels.

The vitamin C connection fared better in a study of twelve asthmatics tested on bronchial constriction brought on by exercise. This is a form of asthma in which sufferers experience chest tightness and wheezing within three to five minutes after exercising, and the condition progressively worsens over the next thirty minutes. All asthmatics have this syndrome to some extent, and in many it's the prominent feature of their disease.

Two New Haven, Connecticut, physicians, Alan Schlesinger and Neil Schachter, gave twelve subjects either a placebo or 500 mg of ascorbic acid on two separate days, six hours or less before exercise. Compared with the placebo, pretreatment with ascorbic acid led to significantly less bronchospasm (rated five minutes after the exercise). Additional measurements of air flow showed the vitamin C to be extremely effective. In this experiment, a larger dose was not tested. But it is likely that this protective effect would have been even greater if several grams of vitamin C had been administered.

Chédiak-Higashi Syndrome and HIE Chédiak-Higashi syndrome is a rare and usually fatal disease characterized by albinism and a bleeding tendency. Frequent and severe infections plague the victim because neutrophils don't migrate to bacteria at a normal rate and can't kill the bacteria they do ingest.

Young children with this syndrome generally die by their fourth year.

Now two children with the disease are living a normal life, outside the hospital, for the first time since their birth. Lawrence A. Boxer of the James W. Riley Hospital for Children is also an Assistant Professor of Pediatrics at Indiana University School of Medicine in Indianapolis. Dr. Boxer has simply been giving these children a daily dose of 20 mg of vitamin C per kilogram of body weight—the equivalent of several grams of vitamin C for an adult. At the time Dr. Boxer and his co-workers reported, the children had been free of infection for nearly two years.

Patients with hyperimmunoglobulin E (HIE) syndrome also have defective neutrophil action. Too, they have high levels of immunoglobulin E (IgE) in their blood—from whence cometh the disease's exotic name. Patients tend to suffer recurrent serious bacterial or fungal infections along with allergic reactions.

Workers at the Marshfield Clinic and Marshfield Medical Foundation, with Freidenberg as senior author, report dramatic clearing of all these signs when 1 gram of ascorbic acid is taken three times daily.

Another HIE patient developed a *Candida albicans* ulcer on his eye. The ulcer responded well to antifungal therapy, but Drs. Foster and Goetzl of the Departments of Ophthalmology and Medicine at Harvard Medical School chose to look beyond the eye and into the HIE. After a thirty-day course of 300 mg of oral ascorbic acid each day, the patient was free of the signs of his disease. Perhaps even more striking, he developed no infections of any kind during a two-year follow-up—while he remained on vitamin C therapy.

Similarly good results in patients with poor neutrophil motility, high IgE levels, and chronic problems with infection have been reported by Anderson and Theron, by Anderson and Dittrich, and by a research team at Italy's University of Genoa Medical School (Rebora, Callegri, and Patrone). In these several studies, anywhere from 1 to 3 grams of oral ascorbate were given daily. The long-lasting "cure" of patients in the Genoa group prompted those investigators to strongly recommend vitamin C for the prevention and treatment of recurrent infections.

Fever Blisters   Known in professional circles as *herpes labialis*, the fever blister is produced by the herpes simplex virus, Type I. It's an almost universal human parasite, living in about seven to nine out of every ten people, and erupting periodically in about forty percent of the population. Stress seems to be the key—any kind of stress, such as psychological factors, sunburn, a dental appointment, illness or surgery, or loss of sleep. Under certain circumstances, the virus overpowers the body's immune system and one ends up with a painful, fluid-filled blister in or around the mouth.

At the National Naval Dental Center in Bethesda, Maryland, three researchers, Terezhalmy, Bottomley, and Pelleu, successfully treated fever blisters (or cold sores) with therapeutic doses of ascorbic acid and water-soluble bioflavonoids. Fifty patients with recurrent herpes labialis were included in the study; results are summarized below.

NO OF PATIENTS	REGIMEN	% DEVEL- OPING BLISTERS	% EXPERI- ENCING MEMBRANE BREAKAGE	DAYS PAIN EXPERI- ENCED	DAYS RE- QUIRED FOR HEALING
20	200 mg ascorbic acid, 200 mg bioflavonoids 3 times daily for 3 days	36	26	1.5	4.4
20	200 mg ascorbic acid, 200 mg bioflavonoids 5 times daily for 3 days	36	26	1.5	4.2
10	placebo (dummy pill of lactose) once daily	100	100	3.5	9.7

German Measles   At the University of Florida College of Medicine in Gainesville, Waldman and co-workers tested C against the rubella virus. Depending on its route of inoculation, the virus may act and respond differently. In the volunteers who received the virus by nose drops, there was a significant reduction in respiratory symptoms and a significantly earlier appearance of serum antibodies (infection fighters) in those who drank one quart of orange juice per day. But the orange juice offered no protection when the virus was injected under their skin.

Hepatitis   Each year serum hepatitis (Type B) strikes an estimated 20,000 to 30,000 people in the United States. For 3000 to 5000 of them, the disease is fatal. Many who do recover suffer from fatigue for a long time.

But some rather startling—and very good—news comes from out West and down South. Robert Cathcart of Incline Village, Nevada, reports what he terms "dramatic recovery" in twenty hepatitis patients. He treated them by having them take vitamin

C to the point of getting diarrhea and then decreasing the dosage slightly. He says "the patient is feeling essentially well in 3 or 4 days" and that "it generally takes about 6 days for the jaundice to clear and in 2 or 3 days the urine returns to normal color."

In Reidsville, North Carolina, a general practitioner has been treating hepatitis victims for many years by using 400 to 600 mg of ascorbic acid per kilogram of body weight (for a 150-pound adult this comes to about 28 to 42 grams.) Klenner reports that his patients are well and back at work in three to seven days.

And from the other side of the Pacific come reports that vitamin C can *prevent* hepatitis. Doctor Akira Murata of the Laboratory of Applied Microbiology at Saga University in Japan studied large groups of patients at Fukuoka General Hospital and Tachiara Hospital. At Fukuoka General, among 150 surgical patients who had undergone transfusions and had received less than 1500 mg of ascorbic acid a day, the incidence of serum hepatitis was 7 percent (11 out of 150 patients). In the 1095 patients who had been given 2000 mg or more of C each day, there was *not one* case of hepatitis. Similar effectiveness was noted at the Tachiara Hospital. So now vitamin C is routinely administered in both these hospitals, and surgical and intensive-care patients receive 6 to 10 grams of ascorbic acid daily for a few days before transfusion and for several weeks afterward.

Leprosy   Leprosy? Yes, leprosy. At the American Leprosy Mission's Leprosy Atelier of the University of Hawaii, Matsuo, Skinsnes, and Chang serendipitously made the vitamin C connection as they were processing biopsies from leprosy patients in Zaire. One patient had been given 1.5 grams of vitamin C per day for 4½ months without receiving any specific antileprosy therapy. The microscopic evidence was startling. The lesion had regressed to a striking degree. More biopsies were examined. Four others who had received the same vitamin supplement along with antileprosy therapy for from seven to twenty-four months showed the same degree of regression. In all five patients, leprosy bacilli had been almost totally destroyed.

How could this happen? Vitamin C is a specific inhibitor of *Mycobacterium leprae*. In addition, ascorbic acid inhibits one of the enzymes that enables the leprosy germ to use nutrients it gets from substances in connective tissue.

Dr. Skinsnes reports that additional trials are now underway, and vitamin C is being given to series of patients afflicted with leprosy.

Pseudomonas Infections P. *aeruginosa* is a microorganism that often establishes a resistant infection in chronically ill or debilitated patients. As a longer life expectancy and more sophisticated medical tools increase this population, ways of combating P. *aeruginosa* gain even more interest.

Counting microbes in sputum is an effective way to evaluate the severity of infection and the response to treatment. In a study where antibiotic therapy was combined with a twice-daily dose of 2 grams of vitamin C, Rawal, McKay, and Blackhall observed a remarkable reduction in the number of live microorganisms, as outlined below.

	WEEKS OF THERAPY				
PATIENT NO.	0	1	2	3	4
1	300,000	3,000	200	0	0
2	20,000	10,000	100	30	10
3	1,000	100	0	100	10
4	4,000	0	0	10	1,000
5	10	1	1	1	1

The investigators' conclusion: the combination of ascorbic acid and antimicrobials has significant therapeutic potential in a variety of chronic infections. This could revolutionize antibiotic treatment. It's for sure that help is needed, because resistant microbial strains develop faster than scientists turn out new drugs.

Rabies This is one of the most dreaded viral diseases known to humankind. It attacks the central nervous system, producing convulsions, paralysis, and an agonizing death.

Obviously one cannot experiment with rabies in people! But, like human beings, guinea pigs cannot synthesize vitamin C and are dependent on dietary sources. So Dr. Banic of the Institute of Microbiology, Medical Faculty, in Ljubljana, Yugoslavia, selected these little animals as his "guinea pigs."

He inoculated forty-eight test animals and fifty controls with a lethal dose of rabies virus. Then, six hours after inoculation, each of the test animals began receiving vitamin C. Intramuscular injections containing 100 mg per kilogram of body weight were given twice daily for seven days. The controls were injected with a saline solution. All the animals were observed for fourteen days.

Of the animals treated with vitamin C, seventeen of forty-eight (35.4 percent) died. But this is only half the death rate among the untreated animals (35 out of 50, or 70 percent). The statistical significance of these frequencies is high (P<0.01).

Although the treatment had no therapeutic effect in the seventeen animals that developed rabies and died, we believe that a larger dose (a guinea pig could tolerate two or three times the dosage given) might have worked. In any event, we hope that this preliminary research will be continued in larger groups of lower animals. We think there is merit in Banic's contention that his "results justify the conclusion that vitamin C is effective in rabies prevention."

Urinary-Tract Infections   Imagine a grain of sand in your eyes. This is something like the irritation that occurs when "loose crystals" are in the urethra. This crystalline phosphate material occurs because the urine is too alkaline to keep these crystals in solution. Microbes also begin to multiply in the alkaline urine. They can't survive in acid urine.

Realizing that ascorbic acid is an effective means of making urine more acid, Stephen N. Rous, Chief of Urological Service at the New York Medical College–Metropolitan Hospital Center, started giving patients 3 grams of vitamin C each day for four days. Complete relief occurred in two to four days. Those patients who reported any recurrence of symptoms were always relieved by a repeat course of ascorbic acid.

Kathryn E. Nickey of the University of Tennessee College of Nursing reports similar success in acidifying the urine of convalescing hospital patients. She found 1000 mg of vitamin C four times a day and 8½ ounces of cranberry juice taken four times daily to be about equally effective. But the combination of the two brought the best results.

THE NOT-FINAL FINAL WORD

W. J. McCormick of Toronto advocates the use of ascorbic acid for *all* infectious disorders. He reports that when 500- to 1000-mg doses are given intravenously or intramuscularly every hour or two, the effects compare favorably with those resulting from antibiotics that are routinely prescribed. McCormick says that "spectacular results" have been achieved in pneumonia, tuberculosis, scarlet fever, pelvic infection, and septicemia.

Dr. Frederick R. Klenner has been using ascorbic acid or sodium ascorbate (orally and intravenously) in all types of viral and bacterial infections for almost forty years. The neutralizing action of vitamin C on a variety of bacterial infections, viral infections, and histamine is, according to Klenner, in direct proportion to the severity of infection and the amount of ascorbic acid given.

All types of pneumonia, bacterial or viral, have been successfully treated by Dr. Klenner with oral doses of vitamin C. His usual schedule is 1 gram per hour for forty-eight hours and then 10 grams each day. Those under ten years of age are given at least 1 gram for each year of life.

The use of vitamin C in the treatment of pneumonia dates all the way back to the late 1930s. It was not uncommon then for pneumonia to occur after prostatic surgery at an incidence of about 12 percent. This was the experience of Slotkin and Fletcher (Millard Fillmore Hospital in Buffalo, New York) until 1939.

They discussed this complication with Dr. Harold W. Culbertson, a prominent Buffalo internist, who explained that, in many cases of nontypical pneumonia, he got excellent results with vitamin C. Following this suggestion, Slotkin and Fletcher "used ascorbic acid (vitamin C) on some 40-odd patients in none of whom have pulmonary signs developed." They achieved this complete victory over postsurgical pneumonia by giving 25 mg of C four times daily until the patient's temperature returned to normal. Even in aged patients they reported (in 1944) that not one death from pulmonary complications had occurred since they began to use vitamin C in 1939.

Who knows how many more infections can be licked with vitamin C? Our guess is that this vitamin will improve the currently prescribed therapy for any infectious disease.

If you take vitamin C prophylactically, there will be less infection in your health future. However, if infection catches you, take more C and consult a nutritionally oriented doctor without delay. The dosages in this chapter are reported to show the vitamin C connection in a variety of infections; they are not prescriptions for you to follow in self-therapy at home.

If you took the quiz at the beginning of this chapter and found that you are prone to infection, you may want to reach for the vitamin C. If it can curb leprosy or prevent hepatitis, it surely ought to help an infected hangnail or that ubiquitous scourge discussed elsewhere in this book: the common cold.

4
Vitamin C:
the Natural Healer

Offstage voice of man in bathroom, howling as if in mortal pain: "Janet, where's the styptic pencil?"

Small boy at breakfast table: "Mommy, that cocoa's burning my mouth!"

Revving up car, woman attempts to adjust sideview mirror and bangs the back of her hand against the half-lowered window. She moans, "Oh, well, one more bruise."

Teenage girl stares wistfully into mirror. Silently she asks: "How can I go to the prom with red cracks in the corners of my mouth?"

Parts of scripts for commercials to accompany the surgery drama unfolded in Chapter 1? No, just some common illustrations of the extent to which Americans are subject to countless small injuries they consider "normal"—not to mention major ones like the trauma connected with surgery.

The Public Health Service published a survey indicating that injuries led to some 130 million physician visits during one recent year. Another year shows a rate of 31.6 persons per 100 who were injured in some way. Among acute conditions requiring medical attention, injuries are a close second to acute respiratory problems. And in nonfederal, short-stay hospitals a recent year saw nearly one out of every two persons undergo surgery at least once during their hospitalization.

How quickly can a person heal? How quickly can *you* heal? Check out your healing status by taking the following quiz. Try to circle your answers in ink so you won't have second thoughts.

Do you bleed unduly if you nick yourself with a razor?	YES	NO
Do you frequently have a burning or scalding feeling in your mouth or on your tongue or lips?	YES	NO
Are your gums frequently sore or tender?	YES	NO
Do you have bleeding gums after brushing, eating, or for no apparent reason?	YES	NO
Do you bruise easily?	YES	NO
Have you noticed that your mouth is frequently dry?	YES	NO
Are you bothered by cracks or raw places at the corners of your mouth?	YES	NO
Do you heal slowly after injury or surgery?	YES	NO
Do you have a stomach or intestinal ulcer?	YES	NO
Have you been avoiding citrus fruit or juice?	YES	NO
Do you avoid taking vitamin or mineral supplements?	YES	NO
Do you have a drinking problem?	YES	NO
Are you diabetic?	YES	NO
Are any of your immediate family or other blood relatives diabetic?	YES	NO
Does any family member or relative have hypoglycemia (low blood sugar) or suffer from alcoholism?	YES	NO
Are you anemic?	YES	NO
Do you smoke?	YES	NO
Do you have cataracts or glaucoma?	YES	NO
Are you taking several prescribed or over-the-counter medicines?	YES	NO
Do you crave sugar, sweetened foods or drinks, or alcohol?	YES	NO

The more YES answers, the greater the likelihood that you recover slowly from injuries (including the physical assault of surgery). Even some people who have no YES answers may be slow healers.

Take heart! You, yourself, can hasten healing or recovery time by as much as 50 to 75 percent. It all has to do with what Walter Cannon many years ago called the "wisdom of the body." Without this natural wisdom, human bodies could not survive.

In this chapter we'll discuss C's input into this body wisdom as that vitamin checks and balances injuries by monitoring our own natural healing process.

HOW IT WORKS

Vitamin C is unique among all vitamins. It serves as a kind of special "glue" that holds cells together. Thus it plays a role in every tissue and organ in the body. A deficiency contributes more damage to more places in the body and creates more biochemical chaos than any other single nutrient.

Consider C's connection to collagen. Collagen is a protein substance that is a critical structural ingredient of blood vessels, the fibrous tissue in scars, and the matrix of hard tissues like bone and cartilage. Defective collagen is chemically tied to deficient vitamin C—megadoses of C encourage the synthesis of more collagen, so that connective tissue is strengthened.

Studies on healthy young adults eating a C-deficient diet (only 5 to 10 mg daily) for periods up to seven months show that wound healing is dramatically delayed. The same subjects showed severe impairment to the tensile strength of healing wounds. This means that the wounds were less able to resist being torn open, and—compared with controls—the deficit amounted to 50 and 60 percent.

Experimental Evidence

A great many traditionally trained health professionals and nutritionists continue to hold the opinion that diet alone can supply all the vitamin C a person needs. But published evidence indicates that supplementation has a profound effect on wound healing.

Gums   As we've mentioned, guinea pigs, like human beings, cannot synthesize vitamin C; they depend on outside sources. A research team at the University of Alabama in Birmingham Medical Center used these little creatures to study the effect of ascorbic-acid supplementation on intraoral healing. Standardized wounds were inflicted, then healing was measured against C intake by injection.

GROUP	DAYS REQUIRED FOR HEALING
No supplement	16.7
2 mg C per day	12.0
20 mg C per day	8.0

Interestingly, 2 mg per day is the amount thought to prevent deficiency in a guinea pig. On the face of it, this certainly seems like an adequate quantity of vitamin C. Yet animals given ten times that amount enjoyed much faster wound healing.

Moving on to people, the researchers experimented with healthy dental students who had acceptable blood levels of ascorbic acid. From each student a small (3 mm) plug of gum tissue was removed and, each day, the wounds were painted with a 1 percent solution of toluidine blue dye, rinsed, and then photographed. Since the dye adheres only to connective tissue beneath the outer layer of gum tissue, it is an effective way of measuring the wound size. That is, one could watch the blue circle become progressively smaller. Healing was judged to be complete when the stain was no longer visible.

After a two-week rest period, a second gingival biopsy was taken, but this time each student received 250 mg of ascorbic acid with each meal and at bedtime for a total of 1000 mg a day, starting with Day 1. The healing time was cut by 40 percent. Other students receiving a 500-mg tablet four times a day (2000 mg daily) showed a 50 percent decrease in healing time as compared with their no-supplementation period. In short, adding just one more gram of C netted an additional 10 percent acceleration in gum-wound healing.

Eyes   Roswell A. Pfister and co-workers of the Department of Ophthalmology at the University of Alabama in Birmingham School of Medicine experimented with rabbits to see if vitamin C could reduce or prevent corneal ulceration and perforation when a caustic chemical was administered to the animals' eyes. Healing time was dramatically reduced with use of 1.5 grams of ascorbic acid daily or by instilling 10 percent ascorbic-acid drops each hour for fourteen hours a day. This daily dose of 1.5 grams is equivalent to 35 grams in a 150-pound human being.

Scarred corneas as the result of bad burns are currently the focus of a project being conducted by the National Eye Institute. Eye-burn patients are receiving oral and topical vitamin C. On the basis of the work done by Dr. Pfister and colleagues, we expect exciting results. Megadoses of vitamin C should accelerate new collagen formation to counteract the rate of degeneration. Although the end result is a scarred cornea, preservation of the fluid-filled chamber behind the cornea and the lens will allow surgical restoration of vision by corneal transplant. In more moderate or mild eye burns, vitamin C treatment should prevent ulceration and allow the cornea to heal without scarring.

Surgery   Vitamin C is used up rapidly during and after surgery. In a study of ten women aged twenty-eight to thirty-five, Shukla administered 500 mg of vitamin C daily from the first to the ninth postoperative day, after instructing the hospital dietetic staff to refrain from giving these patients any citrus fruits or juices. Plasma levels of vitamin C continued to drop even though the patients were receiving supplements, although the rate of decline leveled off.

In another experiment involving sixty-three surgical patients, postoperative ascorbic-acid levels were assessed by measuring the amount in white blood cells (leukocytes). Irvin and his colleagues found a 42 percent reduction by the third postoperative day.

Both these experiments indicate that under certain stressful conditions such as surgery, there is considerable added depletion of vitamin C throughout the body. We are convinced that surgical patients need ascorbic-acid supplements—and in considerably greater quantity than Dr. Shukla used.

But our conclusion is hardly novel. More than four decades ago Alan Hunt, a surgeon at St. Bartholomew's Hospital in London, reported that wound disruption had been reduced by about 75 percent since the hospital adopted routine administration of ascorbic acid in all abdominal-operation patients. The standard regimen was 1000 mg daily (in divided doses) for three days before surgery, then 100 mg daily thereafter, except in the event of certain complicating factors, in which case the dosage was upped.

Back in the same era, Bartlett, Jones, and Ryan of Massachusetts General in Boston reported how from 100 to 1100 mg of vitamin C increased tensile strength of thigh wounds in a sixty-two-year-old man. The higher supplement produced a threefold improvement in the skin and a sixfold increase in nearby connective tissue. This is of special interest because the man showed no *clinical* evidence of vitamin C deficiency—just a plasma ascorbic-acid level of only 0.09 mg. But such a level of deficiency is no news to us. In checking plasma ascorbic-acid levels in seemingly healthy dental students, each year we find that from 10 to 20 percent show levels in the range of 0.00 to 0.20 mg. "Normal" is generally regarded to be 0.60 mg percent; milligram percent (mg %) is a unit of measurement reflecting content of a substance in 100 cc of blood.

Shock, all too frequently an accompaniment to surgery, has also been linked to lack of vitamin C. Way back in the 1940s, Harry N. Holmes, Emeritus Chairman of the Department of Chemistry at Oberlin College in Ohio, made the vitamin C connection by noting that C could decrease the fragility and permeability of capillaries. It is plasma loss from these small blood vessels that can induce shock.

At Dr. Holmes's suggestion, Harold G. Kuehner of Mercy Hospital in Pittsburgh started using 2000 mg of intravenously administered vitamin C before and after surgery in fifty seriously ill patients subjected to major abdominal operations: gastric resections, complex gall-bladder and liver surgery, rectal and bowel resections. He reported to Holmes "a more vital convalescence with less serious complications or sequellae than 50 such cases which were operated on without the aid of vitamin C." Kuehner then tested the effectiveness of ascorbic acid in accidental trauma, giving 500 mg orally to injured miners as soon as possible after their accidents. He concluded: "I am thoroughly satisfied that there is betterment in these cases as compared with similar ones not given vitamin C. When they reach the hospital we seem to be able to go ahead with vital procedures indicated more readily than when we were not using vitamin C."

In his second paper, Holmes reports that Dr. George M. Curtis of the Ohio State University School of Medicine found that "there is now little doubt of the value of vitamin C in the prevention of [surgical] shock."

What would happen if all surgical patients could be discharged in one-half of what is now considered the normal healing time? You will recall the experiment with dental students, in whom 2000 mg of vitamin C a day produced a 50 percent reduction in healing time. More evidence in that direction comes from Ved M. Khosla and J. Edward Gough of the Department of Oral Surgery, University of California, San Francisco Medical Center. They evaluated the management of post-extraction third molar (wisdom tooth) sockets and found that the experimental group given vitamin C and B complex experienced a much better rate of socket healing (in addition to less pain).

So far no one has demonstrated, on a wide-scale basis, that 2000 mg per day is the right amount of supplementation and/or that it will hasten healing time by exactly 50 percent. But no longer can either health professionals or the public ignore the importance of vitamin C to the pre- and postoperative course of patients faced with surgery.

Pressure Sores (Decubital Ulcers) A certain kind of ulcer— sometimes called a "pressure sore" or, more popularly, a "bed sore"— frequently develops in people who are confined to bed or a wheelchair for extended periods of time.

In two paraplegics whose pressure sores were biopsied before and after the daily administration of 1000 mg of ascorbic acid for five and ten days, Hunter and Rajan observed vastly improved collagen formation.

In 23 percent of the ninety-one paraplegic patients studied by Burr and Rajan, leukocyte content of ascorbic acid was found to be low. But those patients with pressure sores had even lower levels. Seven of these patients were given 500 mg of ascorbic acid twice daily for three days. Biopsies showed a definite increase in collagen formation, which would make the patients more resistant to formation of such sores.

A team at the Manchester Royal Infirmary and the University Hospital of South Manchester in England, headed by T. V. Taylor, conducted a double-blind (neither party knows) controlled trial on twenty surgical patients suffering from pressure sores. Ten received tablets containing 500 mg of ascorbic acid twice daily and ten were given tablets containing no active ingredient (that is, a placebo).

The treatment group showed a sharp rise in leukocyte vitamin C level. Other factors were kept constant (such as beds and mattresses, hospital diet, local treatment of the pressure sore). Photographic techniques were used to measure reduction in size of the ulcers, and as can be seen below, the differences are noteworthy.

PLACEBO GROUP (% REDUCTION)	VITAMIN C GROUP (% REDUCTION)
50	81
54	72
4	87
60	87
22	21
39	90
45	100
14	100
60	100
80	100

The average reduction for those receiving the placebo for a month was 42.7 percent. Twice as much healing occurred in the vitamin C group—an average of 84 percent. Analysis of these figures showed a very significant statistical difference ($P < 0.005$). In fact, four of the ulcers had completely healed before the month ended. (The usual time is three to four months.)

More recently, Silvetti and co-workers at the Tissue Reconstruction Institute of Bethany Methodist Hospital in Chicago had remarkably good experience with the *topical* application of vitamin C in combating bed sores (as well as severe burns). In thirty patients with sores that had festered for two months to several years, daily application of a preparation containing vitamin C caused the smaller lesions to heal in four to eight weeks without grafting. Noticeable improvement and decrease in ulcer size were observed on a daily basis, and wound infection was completely eradicated in twenty-four to forty-eight hours after treatment. Larger wounds accepted skin grafts and then also healed in record time.

The Silvetti team says that the sores had not healed earlier because *the necessary nutrients required for new tissue formation weren't circulated to the site of infection.*

Since vitamin C has induced such impressive healing acceleration of pressure sores, we believe it may also act to prevent their occurrence. The only reason we can't be absolutely sure is that no one has tried to do this in a scientific experiment. We hope this is a gap that will soon be filled.

Hereditary Disorders   Seemingly non-C factors such as heredity can play a role in an individual's susceptibility to certain diseases. However, even here, there's a vitamin C connection.

Thalassemia is a hereditary hemolytic anemia that tends to strike people of Mediterranean origin. It plays havoc with hemoglobin (the oxygen-carrying element in red blood cells) and is characterized by an abnormal incidence of leg ulcers. If the person suffers a mild form of thalassemia that's compatible with survival into adult life, these leg ulcers become a major disability and—because of recurrent infections—can pose more of a problem than the anemia.

Scientists at Maadi Military Hospital and St. Thomas' Hospital in London, with Afifi as principal investigator, designed a study to see if vitamin C would help heal leg ulcers in thalassemia. Eight patients with the same form of the blood disease and with from two to four leg ulcers of at least two years' duration were chosen from two related families.

The subjects showed no evidence of C deficiency; they had all been receiving a good mixed diet. They were instructed to continue their normal antiseptic dressing procedures and to raise their legs to a horizontal position for fourteen hours each day (including sleep time). In the team's elegant double-blind, cross-over study, each patient in Group I (four patients) received 1

gram of effervescent ascorbic acid three times daily for eight
weeks, then 3 grams of a placebo effervescent tablet each day for
the second eight-week period. Group II were given these preparations in the reverse order. Results can be summarized as follows:

1ST EIGHT WEEKS

Group I (14 ulcers)   7 completely healed, 5 partially healed
Group II (12 ulcers)   4 partially healed

2ND EIGHT WEEKS

Group I   4 additional complete healings
Group II   9 completely healed

Obviously Group I enjoyed a carryover from their vitamin C regimen. All differences were statistically significant ($P < 0.01$). Since
these high doses of ascorbic acid were effective even in patients
who supposedly had acceptable vitamin C intake, we feel these
findings lend additional weight to the evidence accumulating that
adding vitamin C can hasten the body's natural healing response.

In addition to hemolytic anemia other hereditary disorders affect substantial groups of people. For example, there is a group of
diseases subclassified under the clinical description of Ehlers-Danlos syndrome. The condition is generally marked by too much
extensibility of the joints, fragile skin, and a tendency to sustain
little tumors of blood in response to small injuries.

Elsas, Miller, and Pinell, working out of the Emory University
School of Medicine and Duke University School of Medicine,
treated an eight-year-old boy with Type VI Ehlers-Danlos syndrome. The collagen in his body had only 10 percent of the normal level of hydroxylysine, a protein building block (or amino
acid). The little boy also had only 17 percent of the normal quantity of the enzyme called lysyl hydroxylase, which utilizes vitamin
C when it synthesizes collagen by incorporating the amino acid
lysine into it.

The defective collagen in this young patient had produced
muscle weakness, lax joints, easily damaged skin, many hemor-
rhagic scars, a high-arched palate, and small corneas. Throughout

his life, many cuts and poor wound healing had combined to create abnormal scar formations. Most of his joints could easily be extended far beyond normal range; the tips of both shoulders could actually touch under his chin.

The child's dietary history indicated a regular intake of about 50 mg of ascorbic acid each day, and urinary and plasma levels of vitamin C were within so-called normal ranges. From various tests, it was concluded that "ascorbate deficiency was not present."

So, almost as if to answer the question "Is more better?," the investigators administered 4 grams (that is, 4000 mg) of ascorbic acid daily over a two-year period. The treatment produced a significant increase in the formation of hydroxylysine. Clinically, there was better wound healing, increased muscle strength, corneal growth, a return of bleeding time to normal levels, and improved lung function. Results suggested that the quality of newly synthesized collagen had greatly improved. Since there was no change in looseness of the child's joints, the researchers concluded that the hydroxylysine was not incorporated into collagen that had been formed earlier.

What if vitamin C had been given to the child from birth? It was known at once that a connective-tissue disorder was present; when he was born, he was abnormally weak, had little muscle tone, and the joints in his arms and legs were very loose. One can only speculate, but it is possible that megadoses of vitamin C might have spared the boy a deformed body and a lifetime of compromised physical activity.

THE BOTTOM LINE

If we were into choking horses—which we're not—we'd say there is enough evidence to choke a horse that vitamin C helps wounds heal. So if you answered YES to *any* of the questions near the front of this chapter; or the next time you bump your hand, nick yourself with a razor, cut your finger along with the turkey; or if you must face a surgical operation, seek out a nutrition-oriented doctor who will prescribe vitamin C. Ask about C when you speak

with your pharmacist, health-food store owner, nutritional counselor, or anyone else who is familiar with the almost miraculous
healing power of ascorbic acid as we've described it in this chapter.

5
The Thermostat in *Your* Energy Crisis

Some of us are old enough to remember when there was no air conditioning. How did we ever survive! Even more Americans are old enough to remember when there was no such thing as an energy crisis. When winters got cold, we simply elevated the thermostat several notches—sweaters were garb we wore out of doors.

It used to be that "everyone talks about the weather, but nobody does anything about it." Now it's more like "everyone talks about the weather, and everybody's doing everything about it." We have central heating, thermal underwear, solar energy, Scandinavian-type fireplaces with special vents, portable electric heaters, and various devices that lend a "modern" touch to age-old systems such as heated stones, steam under pressure, or simply the layering of clothing. When it's hot we have not only air conditioning but also air coolers, fans, vented clothing, cold showers, and other amenities our forebears lacked.

But sometimes technology takes its toll. In really hot climates, the parking lot of a shopping mall can be the hard bed for unconscious bodies of people who couldn't quite make it from the air-conditioned car to the air-conditioned supermarket or back.

How well do *you* fare when the temperature soars, with no promise of relief?

Do you frequently postpone outdoor activities such as
    weeding or engaging in sports?   YES   NO
Do you seem not to sweat enough whether exercising or
    lounging about?   YES   NO
Are you plagued by skin rashes in warm weather?   YES   NO
Do you experience a lot of fatigue when summer's heat
    sets in?   YES   NO
Does exercise of any sort (working or playing) leave you
    exhausted?   YES   NO

Then, when the tables are turned and winter takes over:

Are you usually uncomfortable when you have to ven-
    ture outside in cold weather?   YES   NO
Do you often have the feeling that not even the thickest
    gloves and boots offer protection against cold hands
    and feet?   YES   NO
Do you find yourself curtailing winter activities you
    used to like (for example, skiing) because you can't
    stand the cold?   YES   NO,

The more YES answers the more likely you are among those
many, many Americans who find themselves unwilling captives
to the weather. In the summertime you may not pass out on the
pavement of a shopping mall, but you are apt to put off doing
anything that requires leaving the artificial coolness of your air-
conditioned home or office.

Help is in sight!

You need look no farther than your medicine chest. Reach for
vitamin C instead of an iced beverage!

Vitamin C? *Again?* Are we putting you on? Not at all! Read
on.

OUTFOXING THE DESERT FOX

Back in World War II a young medical-corps captain outfoxed the Desert Fox. Two American contingents were being readied to take on Rommel at a time he had been rolling his tanks across the desert with impunity.

One set of troops—inland, closest to Rommel—were beset with extreme heat exhaustion. The men were judged worthless for battle. The other contingent was training in temperatures that were virtually the same. But these men were closer to the coast, with almost unlimited access to fresh citrus fruits. They were considered combat-ready.

The young captain took action. He requisitioned cases of vitamin C tablets. Once they were distributed to the heat-felled soldiers, sick calls for heat exhaustion ceased.

There have been many stories and movies about how General Rommel was "really" defeated. We like to think that vitamin C was on the side of the Allies!

In any event, Dr. G. A. Poda, a physician with E. I. du Pont de Nemours and Company, remembered having read an article about this wartime experience. It proved lucky for Dick (not his real name), a traveling salesman who almost lost his job.

Air-conditioned cars weren't common in the summer of 1951. Dick had suffered a heat stroke the summer before, and now he was becoming extremely weak whenever the temperature rose above 85° F. In fact, his weakness was very much like being in shock. He felt he could no longer cover his territory and sought help from Dr. Poda in Aiken, South Carolina.

Recalling the story of outfoxing the Desert Fox, Dr. Poda decided on a course of 100 mg of ascorbic acid three times a day. Even though temperatures inside Dick's car stayed between 90° and 105° F, the salesman was able to resume his regular working hours. Dick was a cured man, except when he forgot to take his vitamin pills. "Anytime he skipped a day," Dr. Poda told us, "he'd have to find himself a shady spot and just sit there—totally washed out. Then, when he resumed taking the vitamin C supplements, he functioned beautifully."

A fluke?

"No way," says Dr. Poda.

Another success story involved a pro tennis player. The man's bouts with recurrent heat exhaustion were so serious he could not teach or play between 10 A.M. and 4 P.M. Dr. Poda prescribed 500 mg of C once or twice daily. The tennis pro returned to his normal schedule.

Convinced vitamin C can do the trick in preventing heat exhaustion, Dr. Poda now recommends ascorbic-acid tablets for his company's employees. He says: "I urge everyone to take 100 mg two to three times a day—when they come to work in the morning, at their lunchbreak, and, if they're going to be active in the evening, another at quitting time. I've been doing this for years, and have yet to see our first case of heat exhaustion." This is so even though "the climate can be wicked. Many of our people work outdoors [and they are] subjected to heat blasts that come as real shockers."

RESEARCH RECORDS

Unfortunately, traditional-minded scientists tend to downgrade empirical or trial-by-error experimentation. So Dr. Poda's experience, even though it was also reported in a highly respected journal of internal medicine, might be snubbed by some professionals.

Fortunately for all of us, there is plenty of additional evidence that vitamin C acts as a thermostat for any internal energy crisis our bodies may be faced with.

The Heat's On

Exhaustion   Workers in America's Southland may have it rough, but South African mines provide a far more drastic working climate. Mine owners have had to initiate all sorts of acclimatization procedures in step-by-step progression. Even so, most new workers suffer severely from the heat.

Researchers from the Industrial Hygiene Division of the Chamber of Mines of South Africa, led by N. B. Strydom, divided sixty new mine workers into three groups: those receiving 250 mg of C daily; those receiving 500 mg daily; and those who took a dummy tablet (placebo). The men then went through the progressive stages of acclimatization in chambers simulating a mine's atmosphere. Various measurements of heat adaptation—temperature, heart rate, amount of perspiration—were recorded, with both C groups showing a clear advantage. For example, rectal temperatures were taken at 0, 1, 2, 3, and 4 hours of exercise each day. The C groups "won" by one full day on the average. And a startling 35 percent of these "winners" adapted in only three or four days, while only one placebo subject did so and some did not make it even in ten days.

Actually, such findings should not come as a surprise. Back in 1939, roughly forty years before Strydom and his associates did their work, W. L. Weaver of Richmond, Virginia, started a See-What-C-Can-Do program. When a Southern rayon plant's primitive air-cooling system broke down in 92° F temperatures and 90 percent humidity, Dr. Weaver decided to test vitamin C under the cruelest of working conditions. He chose to administer 100 mg of ascorbic acid each morning to men in the maintenance group, people at high risk because of their hard physical labor under especially stressful conditions. For instance, they might have to work in ceiling crawl spaces where temperatures frequently remained over 100° F The other group was made up of operators who performed only moderate physical work. Both groups continued to take the salt and dextrose tablets all workers received routinely.

None of the men who took vitamin C developed symptoms of heat exhaustion; in the other group—even with their lighter work load—nine men did. So a factory-wide program was initiated; every worker was educated to take daily supplements. In 1947 Dr. Weaver reported *no* instances of heat exhaustion since 1938, when the plant had had twenty-seven such cases.

Prickly Heat To the nonsufferer, prickly heat sounds like an innocuous enough little ailment. But the tiny pimples can close pores, causing an abrupt elevation of body temperature. Moreover, the intense itching and sensations of "crawlies" and burning can interfere with sleep and concentration. Secondary infection is common when victims scratch themselves.

During World War II, prickly heat in its more formidable forms—miliaria, miliaria rubra, lichen tropicus, sudamina—caused great anguish to troops in the South Pacific. Just as the young physician-captain outfoxed Rommel in Africa, Robert L. Stern, an enterprising Army doctor in the South Pacific theater, treated heat-rash victims with 300 to 500 mg of ascorbic acid given on a daily basis. The itching cleared and the rash subsided, usually within thirty minutes. The soldiers remained symptom-free for six to twenty-four hours.

Back home, two physicians, Ralph E. Pawley and Charles A. Berry, tested this vitamin C connection during the summer of 1950. Practicing in a small community bordering on a California desert, Pawley and Berry were beset with patients complaining of prickly heat. The doctors gave 500-mg oral doses of C to adults and older children and 100 mg to infants eight pounds or under. Itching was relieved and the rash was cleared in every case. Significantly, none of the victims showed clinical signs of vitamin C deficiency and the same held true for Dr. Stern's soldier patients.

But the full weight of a journal specializing in dermatology came with the report by Hindson and Worsley. Dr. Hindson was first drawn to vitamin C as a treatment for prickly heat while he served as a dermatologist at the British Military Hospital in Singapore. It was a happy accidental finding. He interviewed an Australian Air Force officer who had suffered severe heat rash in the groin area. He had scratched himself raw, provoking a secondary infection. (Medical diagnosis: intertriginous dermatitis secondarily infected with monilia). The painful rash had lasted for a year, resisting all forms of therapy.

Then the man caught a cold and took 1000 mg of ascorbic acid each day for a week. During that week, his heat rash cleared up. On a wise hunch, Dr. Hindson placed the officer on 1000 mg (1 gram) of vitamin C as the sole treatment for the dermatologic condition. Just ten days later, examination showed a normal groin area.

Hindson decided to experiment—first with five children given vitamin C in amounts equivalent to the milligrams per body weight of the Air Force officer. He then worked with thirty children who had suffered repeated attacks of heat rash. Of the fifteen youngsters given ascorbic acid for two weeks, fourteen were entirely rash-free or improved. Of the fifteen children given dummy pills, only four children showed any improvement. For the next two months, all thirty were given vitamin C and no further rash was noted.

Then, working with an associate at the hospital, Hindson used plastic bandages to wrap one arm each of thirty-six apparently healthy servicemen for forty-eight hours. Vitamin C (1 gram daily) was given to eighteen subjects, and a placebo to the eighteen others.

One week after the arms were unwrapped, seventeen placebo subjects still showed sweat-gland fatigue (hypohidrosis)—ten of them to a marked degree. But in the ascorbic-acid group only two subjects showed hypohidrosis—and then only to a mild degree.

This experiment is important to understanding *how* vitamin C might work against prickly heat. With excessive sweating, certain heat-exhausted enzyme systems tend to blank out. One of these, the succinio-dehydrogenase system, is known to be the first to go. It's believed that vitamin C may then "take over" that enzyme system's role in blocking or reducing sweat-gland fatigue, thus minimizing or eliminating sweat-influenced heat rashes.

Jack Frost's In

Early research on rats and guinea pigs showed that high levels of vitamin C can counteract the cold. Then monkeys were used. A group given 325 mg of vitamin C before being exposed to sub-freezing temperatures fared far better than the group given only 25 mg daily. The latter animals also experienced more tail frostbite.

Thus, human beings bound for snow might want to think not only of warm pants but also of popping about 4000 mg of vitamin C per day. That's the human equivalent (given 150 pounds of weight) of the amount given the monkeys who proved more resistant to the cold.

How about research with people?

Professor M. Nakamura and co-workers from the Faculty of Medicine, Hirosaki University in Japan, decided to enlist some volunteers on the theory that what's good for monkeys is good for medical students. They administered 200 mg of ascorbic acid daily for seventeen days to twenty healthy young adults whose diets furnished about 80 mg of ascorbic acid each day of the testing period. By measuring skin temperature before and forty minutes after exposure to cold (5° C or 41° F), the investigators conclusively showed that the C-supplemented subjects showed higher skin temperature.

Livingstone observed the effect of 2000 mg of vitamin C each day on subjects whose middle left fingers were immersed in ice water for thirty minutes. Other left-middle-finger temperatures were recorded for subjects standing in −23° C (−9° F) atmospheres, wearing Arctic clothing but with their hands bared. Results with C were so positive that Livingstone recommends that vitamin C supplements be placed alongside military rations for cold-weather maneuvers. This suggestion proved out when eleven troops stationed in the Arctic were fed diets rich in C-carrying fruits and vegetables. When these soldiers first submerged their middle left fingers in ice water, the average temperature was 37.4° C (99.3° F). After two weeks of working in subfreezing cold—but with vitamin C-rich diets—the men showed an average finger temperature of 42.8° C (109° F).

Reporting at an international symposium held in Novosibirsk, Siberia, a group of Soviet scientists headed by V. M. Krasnopevtsev confirmed that large quantities of vitamin C are needed for effective adaptation to the cold of the extreme north.

HOW DOES IT WORK?

We see plenty of evidence for vitamin C's providing protection against the heat of summer and the cold of winter. But *how* does our "miracle vitamin" do this?

When the mercury soars, the body's coping mechanisms rush to the defense: blood vessels dilate, the heart pumps mightily, sweat pours from the skin. All these actions are set off by hormones, including those secreted by the adrenal gland, a kind of "operation control" that houses more vitamin C than any other tissue in the body. When relentless hot weather depletes supplies, the adrenal gland is less able to produce its various temperature-regulating responses. So body temperature rises, remains raised, and we are subject not only to "the summer blahs" but also to heat exhaustion or even heat stroke.

In extreme cold, blood vessels also dilate. It's called a *cold-induced vasodilator (CIVD) response*. Vitamin C acts to keep blood flowing, particularly to our cold-susceptible extremities.

We live in an era of modern technology that provides us with means of escaping seasonal fluctuations in temperature. But hovering close to an air conditioner or a heater does more than limit our lifestyles. It may also contribute to further dampening natural resistance. So it makes a lot of sense to heed vitamin C's connection to combating the effects of temperature extremes.

6
Pain and Vitamin C

Is there really such a thing as *enjoying* pain? That's a dispute we'll happily dodge—except to remind readers of an interesting fact. Just within recent years, on the other side of the Atlantic, a member of *la famille de Sade* sought to clear the name of his famous (infamous?) ancestor.

Certainly the vast majority of people regard pain with dread. According to statistics compiled by the Public Health Service not too long ago, 94 million Americans over the age of twenty use aspirin and 29 million of them take it regularly—that is, once a week or more often. That's roughly three-fourths and one-fourth of our adult population.

And that's just *aspirin*. Prescribed pain killers, not to mention the increasing array of over-the-counter preparations, account for even larger numbers of people who pop pills for pain.

If you started this book with the introduction and have read straight through, at this point you probably won't be surprised to learn what natural food ingredient has been found effective against pain. Yes, it is vitamin C!

C's CONNECTION WITH PAIN

Muscle Pain and Stiffness

Rare indeed is the adult who hasn't experienced sore, tender, aching muscles after engaging in unaccustomed exercise or manual labor.

Back in the 1960s, James C. Greenwood, Clinical Professor of Neurosurgery at Baylor University's College of Medicine, routinely gave patients with vertebral-disk problems 250 mg of ascorbic acid four times daily. He discovered that these patients enjoyed greatly reduced muscle soreness when they returned to vigorous physical activity. If they neglected to take their tablets, muscle soreness returned. When they resumed taking the vitamin C, muscle soreness disappeared.

The same effect was observed by I. H. Syed in London, England. He described the phenomenon this way: "that muscle stiffness and pain which arises after exercise or an unaccustomed work could be prevented and treated by taking massive doses of ascorbic acid."

Syed's "massive doses" amount only to 500 mg of vitamin C before exercise and 400 mg afterward, along with plenty of fluids. His experience is that this quantity is generally sufficient to prevent stiffness and pain the following day. However, if some discomfort does occur, Syed recommends another 400 mg of ascorbic acid (with fluids) first thing in the morning and one or two doses of 200 mg every two hours if required.

A unique and well-controlled study of vitamin C and muscle pain was designed by Gupte and Savant from the Department of Anaesthesiology, Tata Memorial Hospital in Bombay, India.

In preparation for esophagoscopy, direct laryngoscopy, and bronchoscopy—nasty-feeling procedures that involve sticking special instruments down people's "throats"—patients are frequently given Suxamethonium, a muscle relaxant. An unfortunate side effect is skeletal muscle pain and stiffness when, in the early postoperative period, patients start to move about.

For their study, Gupte and Savant selected 125 patients (mean age, forty-six) who would each receive a 500-mg tablet of vitamin C twice daily on the day before the examination, the day itself, and the day after. They were instructed to chew the tablets before swallowing them. A control group of 115 patients (mean age, forty-three) was subjected to the same kinds of examination, but minus the ascorbic-acid supplement.

Of the 125 patients who took the vitamin C, only 15 (12 percent) complained of pain—10 "mild" and 5 "severe." In the control group of 115 patients, 42 (36.5 percent) complained of muscle pain—5 "mild" and 37 "severe." All this amounts to a percentage of pain that was threefold higher in the control group, with an eightfold difference in severity. Statistically analyzed, these differences proved to be highly significant.

The same investigators used high doses of vitamin C to reduce or eliminate muscle pain and stiffness in "normals" subjected to strenuous activity.

How Does It Work? Gupte and Savant think that—both with Suxamethonium and unaccustomed exercise—injury to the wall of muscle cells causes the pain, and that ascorbic acid protects against this kind of injury by a mechanism as yet not fully understood. Possibly vitamin C helps detoxify the muscle metabolites that are produced during exercise, enhancing their excretion by diuretic action (making one "have" to urinate).

Dr. Syed theorizes that since vitamin C nourishes the inner lining of capillaries—the smallest vessels in the arterial chain—it may prevent damage to or rupture of these tiny vessels, thus preventing muscle pain.

Low-Back Pain

Since 1975, there have been about 37.5 million visits yearly made to orthopedists. And that does not include visits by orthopedists to hospital in-patients or the nearly one million patients being attended by chiropractors. No figures show exactly how many of these complaints concern low-back pain, but the disorder is known to be one of the most common orthopedic problems.

In our discussion of muscle pain, we mentioned that Dr. Greenwood had started giving vertebral-disk patients vitamin C on a routine basis. He had initially experimented on himself when severe lumbosacral (low-back) pain became increasingly disabling. Once an avid golfer, Dr. Greenwood found that hitting about forty practice golf balls would cause him several days of disability. He began taking 100 mg of ascorbic acid three times a day. Within four months, his back pain was gone and he could exercise freely with very little difficulty. For the next three months, he stopped taking the supplements and his "bad back" returned with a vengeance. Once he resumed taking the vitamin C, the low-back pain disappeared.

Dr. Greenwood related his experience to an orthopedic surgeon, Paul Harrington. Dr. Harrington persuaded him to stay with the C and increase the dosage to 250 mg four times a day— the level he recommended to his own "bad-back" patients and which he himself was taking for back-pain relief.

Returning to his own patients who had early disk lesions and who were experiencing simple lumbosacral pain or sciatic-nerve problems, Greenwood prescribed 750 to 1000 mg of vitamin C daily. Even patients with severe disk involvement thought to require surgery were given short trials of C therapy; a few of them recovered without the surgery. All postoperative patients were told to take 500 mg of C each day for an indefinite period of time, increasing the dosage to 750 or 1000 mg when there was any discomfort.

Summarizing his experience with more than 500 patients, Greenwood notes that "a significant percentage with early disk lesions were able to avoid surgery." He also reports that "the number of reoperations on the same patient for recurrence at the same level or a new disk lesion at a different level was greatly reduced."

How Does It Work?   In an earlier chapter we described how vitamin C is vital to the formation of collagen, that gluelike protein substance that supports bone, cartilage, ligaments, tendons, and other connective tissue. Dr. Greenwood is convinced of C's importance in maintaining or repairing the integrity of intervertebral disks. He also believes—as we do—that the optimal level of C intake is considerably higher than the so-called RDA of only 60 mg.

Bone Pain

Make no mistake about it, fracturing a bone is painful! Some children, teenagers, and young adults are afflicted with a bone disease called osteogenesis imperfecta—Greek-Latin medicalese for imperfect formation of bones. In its less lethal form, the disease displays considerable fragility of bones; victims are apt to fracture easily.

Winterfeld, Eyring, and Vivian, three investigators from the Department of Orthopedics at Children's Hospital in Columbus, Ohio, and the Department of Nutrition, School of Home Economics at Ohio State University, worked with ten osteogenesis imperfecta patients ranging from five to twenty-seven years of age. They administered 1000 mg of ascorbic acid each day for a period of three months. At the end of the three months, retention levels ranged from 255 to 612 mg daily—intake minus urinary excretion. Only five fractures occurred, compared with the pretest rate of from twenty to twenty-two.

Encouraged by these results, one of the researchers, Edward J. Eyring, collaborating with Diann Kurz, selected another experimental group of thirteen patients ranging from newborn to fifteen years of age.

Eight patients received a 250-mg tablet of ascorbic acid four times each day. A control period equal to the vitamin C supplementation period allowed for comparison in number of fractures; these data are summarized below.

SUBJECT NUMBER	AGE AT START OF STUDY	MONTHS ON STUDY	FRACTURES DURING CONTROL PERIOD	FRACTURES DURING STUDY
1	6 (M)	40	32	10
2	8 (M)	40	14	5
3	15 (M)	36	2	1
4	10 (F)	31	4	1
5	10 (F)	42	14	2
6	11 (F)	25	10	3
7	14 (F)	21	1	0
8	6 (M)	10	3	1

Since Subjects 3 and 7 were studied after puberty, when a decrease in fracture rate is generally experienced, the study-period decline is less sharp than with younger children.

The five remaining subjects had no control period: three were placed on 250 mg per day right after birth; a one-year-old baby was given 600 mg of vitamin C each day; the five-year-old child got 1000 mg daily. Results for these very young children follow.

SUBJECT NUMBER	AGE AT START OF STUDY	MONTHS ON STUDY	FRACTURES BEFORE STUDY	FRACTURES DURING STUDY
9	newborn	17	20 (at birth)	2
10	newborn	18	3 (at birth)	2
11	newborn	43	2 (at birth)	0
12	5	40	6 (during the year prior to study)	2
13	1	31	4 (since birth)	2

In addition to showing a decrease in fractures despite increased physical activity, those subjects able to express themselves verbally also described having much more energy and stamina while they were taking ascorbic acid. Physical activity of eight of the thirteen subjects—Numbers 2, 3, 4, 8, 10, 11, 12, and 13—is described by their parents and physicians as "completely normal."

Vitamin C cannot cure this hereditary bone disorder, but it certainly appears to have a lot of potential for controlling bone deformities from multiple fractures and for preventing severe growth retardation. Perhaps larger doses would yield even better results.

Ascorbic acid's effectiveness in relieving the bone pain of osteogenesis imperfecta prompted a group in England at the Department of Biochemistry, University of Surrey, to probe its use in Paget's disease. Paget's disease (osteitis deformans) is a metabolic bone disorder characterized by deformity and severe pain. The deformity results from resorption and formation processes that occur too frequently and too "wildly." The pain stems from nerve compression.

Headed by T. K. Basu, the Surrey researchers used pain and x-ray verification of the disease as criteria for patient selection. The sixteen subjects who met these requirements were given 3000 mg of oral ascorbic acid each day for two weeks. For those who had not experienced complete relief of pain, treatment was switched to 160 units of porcine calcitonin (a thyroid hormone taken from pigs) for as long as was clinically necessary. Results are summarized below, with 0 = "no change," 1 = "partial relief," and 2 = "complete relief."

AGE AND SEX	SITE OF PAIN	DURATION OF PAIN (YEARS)	RELIEF OF PAIN	
			ASCORBIC ACID	CALCITONIN
85M	knee, legs, spine	5	2	
81M	lower back	15	2	
75M	knee, back	9	2	
78F	back, knees, hips	4	1	1
76F	knee, leg	5	1	1
69F	leg	1	1	1
62M	back, leg	5	1	2
78M	leg, knee	11	1	2
81M	neck, back	4	0	2
61M	back, groin	8	0	2
64M	back, groin	10	0	1
78F	back	10	0	1
85M	buttock, leg	2	0	1
81F	legs, ankle	6	0	1
74F	leg, knee	11	0	0
72F	knee, hip	5	0	0

Within five to seven days after starting the ascorbic-acid treatment, three patients claimed complete relief of pain. Therefore, they did not receive calcitonin. They continued to be pain-free—even the subject who had suffered low-back pain for fifteen years. Five reported partial relief of pain while on ascorbic acid; three of these patients did not improve when switched to calcitonin and two did.

In summary, 50 percent of the subjects had complete or partial relief from pain after two weeks of the 3000-mg vitamin C regimen. Possibly higher doses over a longer period of time would have worked even better. We'll have to wait for further research. In the meantime, since calcitonin is quite expensive and there are no contraindications for adding ascorbic-acid supplements, a combination approach might be effective for certain patients.

In any event, as Basu and co-workers put it: "If pain can be alleviated or abolished by cheap easily produced drugs which can be taken orally, like ascorbic acid, this is to be preferred to embarking immediately on an expensive course of injections."

How Does It Work? As mentioned in the section on low-back pain, vitamin C is known to be essential for the formation of collagen, the protein matrix of bone. It also acts on blood vessels, areas of inflammation, and nerves that convey sensations.

Cancer-Induced Pain

One of the horrors of terminal cancer is intense pain. This pain, produced by neoplastic tissue's encroachment on vital organs and the nervous system, as well as within bones, is so intense and so constant that morphine and other addictive narcotics are usually prescribed.

But, more than a decade ago, a dramatic breakthrough was announced by Cameron and Baird from the Vale of Leven District General Hospital in Dunbartonshire, Scotland. They found that daily intravenous injections of 10 grams (10,000 mg) of sodium ascorbate relieved the pain in terminal cancer patients. In five patients on a heavy morphine regimen for the control of pain from metastasis ("spread") to several bone sites, four were able to stop using the narcotic within a few days after the vitamin C injections were started. Complete pain control was maintained with the vitamin C alone, and no withdrawal symptoms occurred (see Chapter 15).

Another group of fifty patients with terminal cancer were studied by Cameron and Campbell. Ascorbic acid was given orally and intravenously in doses of 10 grams (10,000 mg) per day. The great majority of patients experienced pain relief. From this and other evidence (see Chapter 10), Cameron and Campbell conclude that vitamin C is of value for pain in terminal cancers of all types.

How Does It Work? Cameron and Baird theorize that vitamin C retards invasive tumor growth within bone, which is usually quite painful. In Chapter 10, you will read a lot about metabolism; chemical interactions between dietary nitrates and ascorbic acid; and other factors that explain why a number of authorities believe vitamin C can be of further help in cancer.

PAIN IN GENERAL

Pain is common to almost all diseases and disorders. So as you go through this book you'll find—in earlier chapters and in chapters to come—many references to illnesses we all know entail pain. But pain itself was the focus of the studies described in this current chapter—and that's the only reason we confined ourselves to the pain of low-back syndromes, bone disorders, and cancer. There is no reason to assume that vitamin C is not also effective in reducing or abolishing pain of many, many other origins.

7
Colds: from Chaos to Conviction

"Folk wisdom" has a curiously tenacious—and somewhat comforting—way of taking over when orthodox medicine gets bogged down in needless, heedless controversy.

The public (ranging from blue-collar workers to biochemists, from file clerks to farmers, from teachers to taxicab drivers) take vitamin C largely to ward off colds.

Doctors—for the most part—usually do not prescribe vitamin supplements and are most definitely not much interested in the common cold! Most researchers want to tackle something more dramatic, like cancer, or more obscure, like kaodzera (a sleeping sickness common in sections of Africa).

This seems to be more than a bit odd because there are an estimated 46 colds per year for every 100 Americans. Annual expenditures for cold medications approach $800 million.

One of the exceptions to the rule is Dr. Edme Regnier, a clinician who trained at Johns Hopkins. After reviewing literally hundreds of approaches to combating the common cold, he concluded that nothing—repeat, *nothing*—has any real effect on the course of a cold except one single entity: vitamin C.

Here's the regimen he recommends:

As soon as you sense a cold coming on, take 750 mg of vitamin C. Every three hours afterward, for a period of three days, take a 625-mg dose. Then, over the next three days, take 400 mg of C every three hours—upping bedtime and morning quantities. Finally, for the last three or four days of treatment, take 250-mg doses every 4 hours.

Dr. Regnier says the treatment will work only if you observe four rules:

1. You must "trap" the cold in its first twenty-four hours. A delay of only one day will reduce your chance of success to less than 25 percent. A longer delay? Don't bother.
2. The vitamin C tablets must be fresh. Pills left over from last year's cold will probably have lost their potency by exposure to light, heat, air, or moisture.
3. Abstain from buttermilk and yogurt, which interfere with absorption of ascorbic acid. Also cut back on meat and fish, which could trigger stomach upsets when you're taking lots of C.
4. Be sure you have a *cold*. Although vitamin C therapy can't hurt you, it's good medicine to know what you're treating.

WHAT *IS* A COLD?

This question leaves both professionals and the lay public in a bit of a quandary because there is no medical agreement on the precise definition of a "cold." There are no clear-cut parameters; for example, when does a "cold" become "the grippe," or when your arms and legs ache and your chest feels heavy, do you have a "cold" or the "flu"?

How Does This Affect Research?

This lack of precise definition has led to some sloppily conducted research in which vastly different conclusions can be drawn.

In his book *Vitamin C, The Common Cold and the Flu*, Dr. Linus Pauling outlined standards he believes should be followed in experiments with vitamin C.

1. Ascorbic acid should be given regularly over a period of time to subjects who were not ill at the start of the trial.
2. Subjects should be selected at random from the larger population.
3. A placebo, a tablet or capsule closely resembling the vitamin C tablet or capsule, should be given to control subjects.

With these stringent requirements in mind, one cannot help being impressed by the following results that were tabulated by Dr. Pauling. These studies show an average decrease in illness of 35 percent in response to vitamin C.

NO.	STUDY	% DECREASE IN ILLNESS PER PERSON
1.	Clegg, McDonald (1975)	8
2.	Anderson, Suranyi, Beaton (1974)	9
3.	Dahlberg, Engel, Rydin (1944)	14
4.	Karlowski, Chalmers, Frenkel, Kapikian, Lewis, Lynch (1975)	21
5.	Anderson, Beaton, Corey, Spero (1975)	25
6.	Coulehan, Reisinger, Rogers, Bradley (1974)	30
7.	Cowan, Diehl, Baker (1942)	31
8.	Anderson, Reid, Beaton (1972)	32
9.	Franz, Sands, Heyl (1956)	36
10.	Elliott (1973)	44
11.	Glazebrook, Thompson (1942)	50
12.	Charleston, Clegg (1972)	58
13.	Ritzil (1961)	63
14.	Sabiston, Radomski (1974)	68

In the five studies (Numbers 3, 5, 7, 9, and 11) in which 70 to 200 mg of vitamin C were given, the average decline in illness-per-person was 31 percent. In the nine remaining studies, 1 gram (1000 mg) was given, resulting in an average illness decrease of 40 percent.

It takes little imagination to assume that, generally speaking, the bigger the dose, the better protection against the common cold. This is an assumption borne out by many experiments.

THE COLD CONNECTION

Way back in the 1930s, considerable work was done that showed the beneficial effects of vitamin C in our struggle with the common cold. Then few serious or full-scale attempts were made to strengthen the connection until 1970. In that year, Linus Pauling's best-seller *Vitamin C and the Common Cold* burst upon the scene, leaving an international controversy in its wake.

Some agreed with Pauling; some did not.

One former skeptic was the late Professor Sherry Lewin, head of the Department of Molecular Biology at London Polytechnic. Plagued by frequent and severe colds, the good doctor had taken to swallowing 50 mg of C each day mostly, as he put it, "to please my wife." One day Mrs. Lewin returned home with the only dosage she'd been able to buy: 1 gram (1000 mg) in an effervescent tablet.

Not wishing to waste the tablets, Dr. Lewin began taking them and noted that the "incidence, severity and duration" of his bad colds were greatly reduced when he took two or three 1-gram doses each day.

Trading on his reputation as a distinguished researcher, Lewin got sixty-nine of his cold-plagued colleagues to test vitamin C. Significant relief came to sixty-four—a better than 90 percent improvement rate.

Convinced he was onto something important, Lewin undertook a long and intensive search into the biologic reasons for the effects he himself had experienced. He traced the functions of vitamin C in the body and published *Vitamin C: Its Molecular Biology and Medical Potential,* a text that offers an explanation for discrepancies in research results. Lewin says that individuals and subgroups have varying capacities to utilize preset levels of C. Even one individual's ascorbic-acid "disposition" can differ, sometimes abruptly, in response to external stress and to internal influences such as enzymatic, hormonal, and metabolic factors. He urges future experimenters to take into account biochemical individuality.

Some *In Vivo* Work

As Professor Lewin found first from his own experience, most researchers agree that "more is better." The Australian physician N. W. Marckwell favors 750 mg as soon as cold symptoms appear, followed by 500 mg every three or four hours. In Nebraska, O. E. Van Alyea opts for 1-gram daily doses, whereas in North Carolina Fred Klenner reports success with amounts ten times that high—10 grams (10,000 mg) every eight to twelve hours in his family practice. An internationally known authority on vitamin C, Cedric Wilson, prefers 2000 mg every four hours—as long as the patient is a woman. He notes that females can maintain normal storage of vitamin C in their leukocytes for about that length of time when they have a cold. Men do not fare so well and may need a higher supplementation.

No one has really answered: "How much is enough?" For example, Robert Cathcart, an orthopedic surgeon, treats colds with as much as 30 to 150 *grams* of ascorbic acid daily—telling people to back off slightly when diarrhea occurs—until the cold is over. Cathcart says that a healthy person can easily tolerate from 10 to 12 grams of C each day; with a cold, that tolerance rises considerably. He even categorizes colds by their gram requirement! Dr. Cathcart says of a 20-gram cold: "he [the patient] has the sniffles and doesn't go to the doctor." When the patient's throat "is so sore that he thinks he has 'strep' and he's aching all over and thinks he has the flu," that is a 100-gram cold.

Cathcart, incidentally, is among those investigators who believe that unless ascorbic acid is taken to the point of causing diarrhea (then you lower the dosage), therapeutic effects won't take hold.

Two Special Studies   Since Linus Pauling published the "special requirements" for studying vitamin C's effectiveness that we listed earlier in this chapter, at least two studies that fit the criteria have been published.

A research group headed by I. McLean Baird of the Department of Medicine, West Middlesex Hospital, Isleworth, England, worked for a three-month period with 353 healthy volunteers seventeen to twenty-five years old. They set about to see what effect small supplements of ascorbic acid would have on the frequency and duration of colds. They used natural orange juice containing 80 mg of ascorbic acid, 80 mg added to synthetic orange juice, and synthetic orange juice alone. Daily dietary intake of C was estimated at 50 mg, so the supplement groups were taking in about 130 mg. All drinks (about 181 ml, or approximately 6 ounces) were administered each morning between 10:30 and 11:30 for seventy-two days.

The vitamin C supplementation significantly increased the number of cold-free subjects. It also led to as high as a 21 percent reduction in total number of cold symptoms.

At the College of Medicine of the University of Florida, R. H. Waldman and three associates worked just with orange juice. All subjects were to be "challenged"—a scientific term that means just what it says—with rhinovirus (a virus associated with the common cold). One week before challenge, seven subjects were given a daily fifteen-ounce glass of orange juice. Another five started taking the juice on the day of challenge. Control subjects were merely given placebo pills.

Of the twelve controls, nine developed bad colds. Of the seven volunteers who began drinking the orange juice a week before challenge, *none* developed any cold symptoms. Of the five who started taking the juice just before challenge, only two developed cold symptoms.

Some *In Vitro* Work

A lot of people seem to feel that experiments with people are most telling. They're less keen about lower-animal studies, let alone experiments done in the laboratory. But the annals of science are filled with studies done *in vitro*, meaning "within a glass" or "observable in a test tube," that eventually see direct application to people.

At Stanford University, Carlton and Patricia Schwerdt incubated cultures of human cells with vitamin C for 2 days and then added a common cold virus (rhinovirus). The vitamin concentration equaled that in a person taking 6 to 10 grams of C daily—an amount that, unsurprisingly to us, did not in any way damage any cells.

According to the Schwerdts, the rhinovirus went through one cycle of growth, and then was inhibited—probably as an effect of interferon's being stimulated by the ascorbic acid. At a period forty-eight hours after the infection procedure, the amount of virus collected from the vitamin C–treated culture was only one-fortieth that from untreated control cells.

CONCLUDING POSTSCRIPTS

In spite of all the positive evidence pointing to vitamin C's connection to the common cold, not everyone has become a "true believer." John L. Coulehan of the University of Pittsburgh School of Medicine reviewed a number of publications and commented: "I agree with Chalmers, who stated in his 1975 review of the controversy, 'I, who have colds as often and as severe as any man, do not consider the very minor potential benefits that might result [from vitamin C] worth either the effort or the risk, no matter how slight the latter may be.'"

As for risk, long before it was found that C is harmless, one daring investigator, S. L. Ruskin, administered one or two injections of 450 mg of calcium ascorbate to over a thousand patients who were getting colds. He reported 42 percent "completely relieved," 48 percent "markedly improved," and concluded that "calcium ascorbate would appear to be practically an abortive in the treatment of the common cold."

As for benefits, a leading researcher in the field, Terence W. Anderson of the Faculty of Medicine at the University of Toronto, echoes what we believe is now majority sentiment. In straightforward, undramatic language, Anderson states: "It is now reasonable to accept that the weight of the evidence is in favor of there being some effect (at least on severity and duration [of colds]) from supplementary vitamin C."

The three of us—coming from three separate scientific disciplines—simply wouldn't be caught with a cold. We'd seize and trap the cold, throwing it out of sight and sound with lots of vitamin C.

8
Pumping C

In the world of nineteenth-century romantic literature, people frequently died of broken hearts. In the last quarter of the twentieth century in America, hearts that are *literally* broken account for an alarming rate of mortality. It's summer. A supposedly healthy man—much given to having frequent medical checkups—drops dead on a golf course. He's fifty-five. Autopsy shows major blood vessels occluded (stopped up) by as much as 95 percent. Much as his widow, children, and little grandson grieved, Jack was by count just one more figure in the long list of statistics concerning Americans with circulatory-system diseases. Such patients won the dubious distinction of ranking first (or principal) among hospital diagnoses in a recent year. Those who survived accounted for an estimated 4.8 million discharges from non-Federal hospitals.

The immediate cause of Jack's sudden death was a massive coronary. The "real" cause was *atherosclerosis*, a common and deadly disease ranked as the number 1 killer in the United States and many other countries. Before we discuss this killer, it might be useful to present thirteen questions adapted from the Cornell Medical Index Health Questionnaire. Scarey as it may seem, throw caution to the wind and answer *honestly*. The more you know about your own cardiovascular system and the more you learn in this chapter about how vitamin C can help "broken hearts," the better off you'll be.

Has a doctor ever said your blood pressure was too high?	YES	NO
Has a doctor ever said your blood pressure was too low?	YES	NO
Do you have pains in the chest or out along the left arm?	YES	NO
Are you often bothered by thumping of the heart?	YES	NO
Does your heart often race like mad?	YES	NO
Do you often have difficulty in breathing?	YES	NO
Do you seem to get out of breath long before anyone else does?	YES	NO
Do you sometimes get out of breath just sitting still?	YES	NO
Are your ankles sometimes badly swollen?	YES	NO
Do cold hands or feet trouble you—sometimes even in hot weather?	YES	NO
Do you suffer from frequent cramps in your legs?	YES	NO
Has a doctor ever said you had heart trouble?	YES	NO
Does heart trouble run in your family?	YES	NO

ATHEROSCLEROSIS: NUMBER 1 KILLER

In the early stages of atherosclerosis, fatty substances are deposited in the inner lining of an artery. Eventually these areas turn into yellowish *plaques* that contain several kinds of fatlike material. This alteration leads to changes in connective tissue and the smooth-muscle cells in an artery's wall. As a plaque grows, blood platelets accumulate, setting the stage for a blood clot (*thrombus*). Growth finally restricts blood flow, eventually causing the "death" of a body part that's supplied or, in more extreme cases, total death itself. This whole sequence of events can take a long time, maybe forty years. The disease is the most common cause of cerebral ischemia (a loss of blood supply to the brain, which can induce a stroke or senility) and myocardial infarction (damage to heart tissue because of a blocked coronary artery).

THE VITAMIN C CONNECTION

Scurvy-like Deficiencies and ECG Abnormalities

The same Scotsman we quoted in Chapter 2, James Lind, discovered there was more to people who are deficient in vitamin C than the lemon-lime connection. In 1757 he wrote: "Persons that appear to be but slightly scorbutic are apt to be suddenly and unexpectedly seized with some of its worst symptoms. Their dropping down dead upon an exertion of their strength, or change of air is not easily foretold."

People don't "drop down dead" without reason. Chances are that Lind's sailors had electrocardiographic (ECG) abnormalities totally unknown at that time but which were readily observed in two scurvy patients examined two centuries later. J. Shafar, a consultant physician to the Burnley and District Group of Hospitals in England, reports that, "After a week of ascorbic acid therapy the tracings reverted to normal." Shafar also studied various cardiac abnormalities in other patients deprived of vitamin C, and Richard H. Follis, Jr., working at the Johns Hopkins Medical School, reported on scurvy's relationship to right-sided heart enlargement.

What if a person does not have diagnosable scurvy but is deprived of vitamin C? In a two-year study conducted at the Sorby Research Institute in Sheffield, England, Sir Hans Krebs fed a no-C diet to ten volunteers aged twenty-one to thirty-four. Two of the subjects became suddenly and severely ill with signs of cardiac attacks that made immediate hospitalization necessary. Their symptoms included intense chest pain, difficulty in breathing, shock, and measurable ECG irregularities.

The Four Seasons

In Chapter 5 we discussed some effects of cold environmental temperatures on blood flow, which might account for seasonal variations in the incidence of ischemic heart disease ("not enough blood"). The subject was studied by three Scottish researchers headed by Dunnigan.

Other British workers, including Constance R. Spittle of the Pinderfields General Hospital, Wakefield, Yorkshire, and B. K. Armstrong's team at the University of Oxford in London, have sought to better define the association between vitamin C and myocardial infarction or ischemic heart disease. Their findings, simply expressed, show a direct connection between summer's greater availability of fresh vegetables and fruit and lowered heart-related mortality rates.

Although E. G. Knox of the University of Birmingham in England was more "directly" concerned with vitamin C and heart attacks or strokes—that is, without reference to season—his findings were similar: the higher the ascorbic-acid intake, the lower the cardiovascular death rates. And in his analysis of data on coronary mortality from the Food and Agriculture Organization and the World Health Organization, Jeremiah Stamler found more of a vitamin C connection than a polyunsaturated fatty-acid connection!

Greater the C, Fewer the Deaths

In spite of the grim mortality rates still reported, there has been somewhat of a decline in heart-attack deaths since the mid-1960s. Some people have attributed this to shifting habits—less cholesterol and saturated fats, increased use of polyunsaturated fats, a lowered consumption of tobacco, more exercise, better control of hypertension, and the availability of more sophisticated coronary care units.

But Dr. Emil Ginter of the Institute of Human Nutrition Research in Bratislava, Czechoslovakia, suggests that the decline may also be related to the substantial increase in vitamin C production/consumption over the past couple of decades—particularly since 1968. He says: "It may plausibly be assumed that the high intake of synthetic ascorbic acid has brought about a substantial decrease in the incidence of marginal vitamin C deficiency and may have thereby contributed to the marked decline in coronary mortality."

In the United States, vitamin C intake has jumped about 35 percent. The United States Department of Agriculture reported per capita consumption rose from 100 mg in 1965 to 135 mg in 1977.

During approximately that same period, we surveyed 832 doctors and their spouses in terms of cardiovascular symptoms and signs (as shown by YES answers to the quiz you just took) and their use of vitamin C. A portion of this group was reexamined annually over a five-year period: 290 subjects increased their vitamin C intake, 88 reduced it.

Three significant findings emerged. (1) There was a low—but statistically significant—correlation between daily ascorbic-acid intake and cardiovascular symptoms and signs. (2) Especially after subjects attended group nutritional seminars, cardiovascular abnormalities declined and use of vitamin C rose. (3) Those 88 subjects who decreased their ascorbic-acid intake showed no statistically significant reduction in cardiovascular signs and symptoms. However, the opposite was true in the 290 subjects who increased their intake of C.

TAKING C TO HEART

Some General Mechanisms

After an acute myocardial infarction, there is a significant fall not only in white blood cell count but also in the level of ascorbic acid in blood plasma. Two researchers at the Department of Medicine, Southern General Hospital, Glasgow, Scotland, Hume and Vallance, explain that when white blood cells respond by rushing to damaged heart muscle, they discharge their stores of C so healing can begin. As new ones replace the ones doing battle, they quickly take up remaining ascorbic acid from the blood plasma. In persons taking only the RDA (recommended dietary allowance) of 60 mg—subjects in the Hume and Vallance study averaged about 51 mg daily—vitamin C is depleted almost to scurvy levels.

This depletion was also noted by Jairo Ramirez and Nancy C. Flowers. White blood cell levels of ascorbic acid were found to be significantly lower in 101 patients ($P < 0.001$) with coronary artery disease as compared with patients free of that disease. This prompted Ramirez and Flowers to theorize that poor ascorbic-acid levels may play a role in both the cause and progression of atherosclerosis.

In Chapter 4, concerning vitamin C's healing capacities, we described work done by Roswell A. Pfister, who found that ascorbic acid will accelerate the healing of damaged corneas in rabbits. The objective was to encourage scar-tissue formation before the wound could rupture. It would be exciting news indeed if this could be applied to myocardial infarctions, so that "blowouts" would become a thing of the past.

Certainly vitamin C has been clearly linked to a decrease in postoperative thrombosis (a dangerous clotting) by a group of surgeons in Manchester, England. Dr. C. A. B. Clemetson of the Methodist Hospital in Brooklyn, New York, maintains that C deficiency produces hemorrhage into body tissues by weakening smaller vessels or capillaries; the weakening then causes intravascular (within-the-blood-vessel) bleeding from the capillary-rich lining of large arteries and deep veins.

Fibrinolysis

Fibrin is the final substance produced during the development of a blood clot. It's a spongelike protein substance that forms a web in which blood cells and platelets are trapped.

If this mechanism runs amuck, a thrombus may form inside an artery or vein. When this happens in one of the major arteries surrounding and supplying the heart, we have coronary thrombosis or coronary occlusion.

A number of scientific studies point up vitamin C's contribution to controlling the formation of fibrin. Arun Bordia and his associates at the Ravindra Nath Ragore Medical College in Udaipur, India, found that a single 1-gram dose of ascorbic acid given to healthy adult subjects produced a 167 percent rise in fibrinolytic (fibrin breakdown) activity within six hours. A 131 percent rise was found in twenty patients with coronary artery atherosclerosis. And in a third group consisting of healthy adults, the same dose blocked the fall in fibrinolytic activity that routinely follows eating a high-fat meal.

In a later report, Bordia describes impressive results in myocardial patients: 1 gram of vitamin C caused a 50 percent greater clot-destroying activity.

Similar results have been reported by Mitiyuki Shimizu's research group at Showa University School of Medicine in Tokyo and by Dr. Constance R. Spittle in England. Spittle commented that if "vitamin C is given as quickly as possible after people are admitted to a hospital with a condition which exposes them to a deep vein thrombosis, they should be protected."

Clot control is extremely important because of the likelihood of an embolus. An embolus, so to speak, is a "thrombus on the loose." It may break off and circulate through blood vessels until it finds one too small to slide through, often in the brain (a stroke) or in the heart itself.

Platelet Stickiness

Platelets are cell-like particles in the blood that help regulate blood clotting. In atherosclerosis, they may cling to the inner lining of damaged arteries; there they release substances that stimulate an overgrowth of smooth-muscle cells. This is the beginning of the *plaque* introduced early in this chapter. As platelets congregate in this new site, they may produce a thrombus that partially or completely blocks the artery.

By "stickiness" we mean the process technically called adhesion or aggregation. Platelets may also stick to each other as they circulate through the body. This is especially apt to happen in veins most distant from the heart, that is, leg veins. Muscle contraction is what forces blood up out of the legs. Inactivity allows pooling of blood so that sticky platelets aggregate in what's called *sludging*. Sludged blood, being thicker, does not circulate properly. If you examine sludged blood under a microscope, you can see clumps of platelets and red blood cells. Just as a rolling snowball gathers more snow, such a clump can continue to pick up more platelets and red blood cells and eventually plug up an artery.

In England, R. D. Eastham of Frenchay Hospital in Bristol and P. R. D. Kent of Pfizer Limited in Sandwich found the highest numbers of sticky platelets in early spring and the lowest number in autumn. This parallels the vitamin C intake from fresh fruits and vegetables we discussed earlier under "The Four Seasons."

C's part in combating platelet stickiness was also investigated by Alfredo Lopez-S of the Louisiana State University School of Medicine in New Orleans. Human platelets were first incubated with increasing amounts of vitamin C. Encouraged by anti-stickiness effects in test-tube experiments, Lopez-S and his colleagues took to working with healthy persons. Simply administering 2 grams of vitamin C for two weeks decreased aggregation of the platelets and significantly increased "lag time" in a biological sequence that leads to platelet stickiness. Lopez-S believes that, in addition to inhibiting adhesion to collagen, vitamin C may stimulate prostaglandin E_1, which blocks platelet aggregation.

Success in reducing platelet adhesion was also achieved by A. K. Bordia at the Indian medical college mentioned earlier in this chapter. Forty male patients with coronary artery disease were divided into three therapy groups: those receiving placebos, 500 mg of C twice daily, or 1000 mg twice daily for six months. Follow-up continued for another two months.

The lower-dose group saw a reduction in platelet adhesion of 10 percent. Patients who received 1000 mg showed a 27 percent decrease, which was statistically significant at the $P < 0.01$ level. When treatment stopped, the stickiness progressively increased to near pretreatment levels.

At the Veterans Administration Medical Center and the Medical University of South Carolina in Charleston, a group headed by K. E. Sargi sought to determine whether vitamin C could be linked to the increased platelet adhesiveness and aggregation found in diabetes mellitus. Both in vitro (test tube) and in vivo (using diabetics as subjects) studies were performed, with results clearly showing that ascorbic acid successfully combats the platelet stickiness common in diabetes. This is of special interest here because diabetics are prone to cardiovascular disease.

Vascular Integrity

Sometimes the turbulence of swiftly moving blood or some other mechanical trauma can cause a permeability or porousness of arterial walls—allowing infiltration of cholesterol and consequent plaque formation. The integrity or soundness of arterial walls thus acts as a deterrent to development of atherosclerosis. This soundness depends largely on vitamin C because that nutrient is responsible for the formation and maintenance of the arterial framework and ground substance. The framework consists primarily of the interlacing fibrous protein called collagen, and the ground substance is a biologic cementing medium that binds the collagen into a sturdy unit. The structural picture is completed by an intercellular "glue" that holds connective tissue, muscle, and innerlining cells together.

To demonstrate how restricting C can contribute to groundsubstance injury, G. C. Willis first worked with guinea pigs. Then, collaborating with Dr. Fishman, he autopsied human aortas (the large artery leading from the heart) for ascorbic-acid contents. Arterial depletion was greatest in areas of the artery subject to extra mechanical stress (such as where they branch or divide). It could also be related to the duration and extent of the victim's illness. Willis and Fishman made note of the fact that a "gross and often complete deficiency of ascorbic acid frequently exists in the arteries of apparently well-nourished hospital autopsy subjects. Old age seems to accentuate the deficiency."

The ocular-burn studies of Pfister and his associates, which we mentioned earlier in this chapter, suggest that a kind of localized scurvy develops at the site of trauma. Richard H. Follis, Jr., of the Armed Forces Institute of Pathology, wanted to see how this condition might be related to an escape or discharge of blood. When he immobilized guinea pigs' knee joints, there was little evidence of scurvy in the C-depleted animals. When the animals' knee joints had to bear their usual share of body weight plus that normally carried by the immobilized joint, hemarthrosis (discharge of blood into a joint) occurred quickly.

How does this fit with "vascular integrity"? The more permeable and porous the blood vessel(s), the more one can expect blood to collect in sites where it shouldn't stay. This may result in a variety of problems that are seemingly unrelated—retinal hemorrhage, small strokes, minor heart attacks, miscarriage from placental hemorrhage, gum inflammation and pyorrhea, retarded wound healing, postoperative pain from the leakage of plasma (which causes edema, or swelling), contact sport injuries, and a tendency to bruise easily.

If scorbutic guinea pigs develop atherosclerosis, will vitamin C reverse the process? Another study by Willis proved it would. How about human beings? Working with Montreal-based research associates, Willis decided to find out by using serial arteriography. This entails injecting a chemical that makes the arteries visible and then taking a series of x-rays. Subjects were divided into two groups: atherosclerotic patients given 500 mg of ascorbic acid three times each day and controls who weren't. In the C-treated group, 60 percent of the subjects showed a reduction of plaque size. In the untreated group, there was *no* reduction in plaque size; in fact, in 50 percent of the controls, plaque size increased.

Anthony Verlangieri, Ph.D., of Rutgers University, identified our C-dependent ground-substance component as chondroitin-4-sulfate. The Director of the Institute for Arteriosclerosis Research at Loma Linda University School of Medicine, Lester M. Morrison, administered chondroitin sulfate A (CSA) to patients with established coronary heart disease. The 120 patients were divided into two equal-numbered groups and studied over a six-year period. The group receiving only conventional treatment was beset by 42 coronary incidents, with 14 fatalities. The group receiving CSA along with conventional treatment had only 6 coronary incidents (4 of them fatal). Statistical analysis showed that there is but one chance in a thousand that this could have occurred "by accident"!

Blood Lipids

A lot of publicity has been given to blood lipids—blood fats that include cholesterol and the triglycerides. Actually, epidemiologic studies show that elevated levels of these substances do not necessarily make one prone to atherosclerosis. As a matter of fact, the disease can develop, and frequently does, in men who show what's considered a normal cholesterol level (less than 250 mg percent).

It's true that an excess of cholesterol can be lethal if atherosclerosis continues unchecked. On the other hand, the substance is vital to cell survival and growth and it is an important component of cell membranes, sex hormones, and steroid hormones.

Cholesterol results from a whole series of interrelated processes, though most of it is synthesized in the liver and small intestine from acetate, an end product of food digestion. Only about 15 to 20 percent can be linked to what is preformed in food that's eaten.

Cholesterol is carried about the body in two ways. Low-density lipoprotein (a fat-protein complex) carries it from where it is synthesized—mainly the liver—out to distant cells. High-density lipoprotein transports it away from the cells and back to the liver. So the more low-density lipoprotein cholesterol (LDL-cholesterol), the more chance of atherosclerotic changes. The more high-density lipoprotein cholesterol (HDL-cholesterol), the less prone one is to atherosclerosis.

This difference is important. For when a straight-line association was made—that is, the less cholesterol (in general) the better—cholesterol-fighting drugs were introduced that, according to the World Health Organization, actually *increased* by 25 percent mortality associated with those diseases (including heart conditions and stroke) for which it was prescribed. Japanese investigators substantiated that it is not good medicine to keep total serum cholesterol levels as low as possible in efforts to avoid coronary heart disease or strokes. Cholesterol is a vital substance with an optimal range; "too low" can trigger disease (possibly cancer) just as "too high" can.

At the Institute for Human Nutritional Research in Bratislava, Czechoslovakia, Emil Ginter unraveled some mysteries about how vitamin C helps regulate body levels of cholesterol. Guinea pigs kept on a mere maintenance dose of ascorbic acid—comparable to American diets that furnish a human being somewhere around the so-called RDA of 60 mg—showed C persisting at very low tissue levels. Their HDL-cholesterol dropped; serum triglycerides rose; and the total cholesterol showed a 30 to 60 percent increase. What happened? Cholesterol could not be converted to bile acids because of inhibited activity of a liver-cell enzyme called cytochrome P-450. So it backed up and went into overload.

Further vitamin C connections (e.g., effects of ascorbate sulfate in seeing that cholesterol is excreted as cholesterol sulfate; seasonal variations and availability of fresh fruit and vegetables; activating the liver to speed up cholesterol's transformation into bile acids, a process that lowers blood cholesterol level; etc.) have been made by Carlos Krumdieck and Charles Butterworth of the University of Alabama in Birmingham School of Medicine; by University of Illinois College of Medicine researchers headed by Oglesby Paul, who did a long-term study of coronary heart disease in employees at the Hawthorne Works of the Western Electric Company; by Caroline Bedell Thomas and associates studying a prison population at the Maryland State Penitentiary; and by a Scottish research team headed by Dr. Fyfe. Other enlightening work has been reported by Sokoloff and colleagues at the Southern Bio-Research Institute at Florida Southern College, Lakeland, Florida, who worked with subjects having "too high" cholesterol levels; and by groups that studied pastoral tribes in Kenya and Bantus from South Africa whose "too low" cholesterol levels (despite high dietary intake) were corrected with C. And let us not neglect to mention in connection with cholesterol and triglyceride levels further pro-C findings by A. K. Bordia in India, Dr. Jennifer Horsey's team in London, and Dr. Constance R. Spittle in Wakefield, England.

Unfortunately, space will not allow us to detail the intricate steps of all these experiments. Our more scientific-minded readers may wish to drop by the nearest university library to check these important reports. For our current purposes, we can best summarize the ascorbic acid–blood lipid connection by returning once again to Dr. Ginter

"In most human subjects with elevated plasma-cholesterol and plasma-triglyceride levels and latent vitamin C deficiency, resaturation of their tissues with ascorbic acid can significantly lower their blood plasma-cholesterol and triglyceride levels. The prevention of latent vitamin C deficiency means, for at least part of the population, the hope of physiological control of hyperlipemia." This means, in short, that vitamin C can prevent an overabundance of fatty substances in the blood, thereby preventing atherosclerosis in millions of people.

WHERE DOES THIS LEAVE US *NOW?*

Powerful spokespersons in the medical establishment seem to be saying that we cannot consider vitamin C as a therapeutic or preventive approach to cardiovascular disease until a lot more research is done.

How much more? How long should we wait?

We believe that more-than-sufficient published evidence exists *now*—and that the public has a right to demand the practical application of this research *now*.

More than two decades ago, G. C. Willis showed that ascorbic-acid deficiency causes atherosclerosis in guinea pigs *even with normal blood cholesterol levels*. The inner lining of arteries was damaged by small hemorrhages caused by the lack of vitamin C; then cholesterol was deposited there—an aberrant form of wound healing with the name "atherosclerosis."

A review of the Russian scientific literature of the 1940s and 1950s, published by Ernest Simonson and Ancel Keys, shows many reports concerning vitamin C, including its use in treating patients with coronary artery disease (with 500 to 1000 mg orally or 300 to 500 mg intravenously). With the authority of his status as member of the Academy of Medical Sciences and Director of the Institute of Experimental Therapeutics in Moscow, Miasnikov said in quite a direct manner: "Ascorbic acid is widely used for prevention and therapy of atherosclerosis."

Exactly what are we supposed to wait for?

If you had a couple of yes answers to the quiz near the beginning of this chapter, or if you otherwise feel at risk for cardiac or cardiovascular problems, don't wait until all the doctors are willing to use vitamin C as a treatment. Seek out a nutritionally oriented practitioner who recognizes that—while all the answers may not be in—*lives* can be saved with vitamin C. We predict that "pumping C" is going to see a lot of action and "the life you save may be your own."

9
Sugar Is Sweet–
Except in Diabetes

If your grandmother had diabetes, her age-peer relatives probably said of her: "She has sugar, you know." This did not refer to
her temperament or her pretty face but rather to the disease
called *diabetes*. The label comes to us from the Greek, meaning
"to siphon or to pass or run through."

The "running through" describes the frequency (and often the
volume) of diabetics' urination patterns. But the old term "having
sugar" aptly enough describes what is technically called *glycosuria;* that is, glucose (a form of sugar) is not properly metabolized
so that it spills over into the urine.

One of the problems in understanding orthodox medicine's
view of diabetes is that even the experts can't reach agreement on
limits of the disease. For example, blood glucose (often called
blood sugar) is frequently measured by the glucose tolerance test.
A high reading suggests diabetes mellitus. But how high is
"high"? When K. M. West surveyed the scene, he found wide
discrepancies. What half the diabetes specialists considered abnormal the other half would classify as normal, meaning "within
physiological ranges." Cause and effect links remain unclear.
And, since diagnostic criteria remain fuzzy, it is not surprising
that therapeutic approaches vary. About all that can be certain is
that when sugar is "high" (whatever that is), doctors seek to bring
it back to "normal" (whatever that is).

Another confusing issue is: How many diabetics are there? Traditionally, it's been held that 1 percent of Americans have it and
they know it. Another 1 percent have it but don't know it. The
latest (and already pretty old!) official estimate dates back to

103

1975—4.8 million persons of all ages have diabetes. Yet a distinguished endocrinologist at the University of Pittsburgh, Thaddeus S. Danowski, says that, during the course of a lifetime, about one out of four Americans "develops diabetes or episodes of hyperglycemia that are indistinguishable from diabetes." Dr. Danowski's figures would mean 25 percent, not 2 percent—although it is somewhat doubtful that most people, including doctors, would consider transient bouts of hyperglycemia as being *really* diabetes.

But if you want to get at least some idea of your *own* risk factors, circle answers to the following questions.

Have you noticed increased thirst?	YES	NO
Has there been an increase in urination lately?	YES	NO
Have you experienced increased appetite?	YES	NO
Are you overweight?	YES	NO
Do you suffer with a dry or burning mouth?	YES	NO
Have you recently required a decided change in your prescription for eyeglasses?	YES	NO
Do you have tenderness of the gums?	YES	NO
Is there a history of diabetes in your family?	YES	NO
Have you lost considerable weight lately?	YES	NO
Have you ever been told that your blood sugar was suspiciously high?	YES	NO
Do you have periodontal disease?	YES	NO
Do you crave sweet foods and beverages?	YES	NO

For the male, you might also answer the following question.

Do you have a problem with impotency?	YES	NO

For the female, try the next two.

Do you suffer with vaginal itching or other signs of a possible infection?	YES NO
Have you had a baby who weighed more than nine pounds at birth?	YES NO

If some YES answers frighten you, don't run for help. You may or may not have what doctors may or may not call *diabetes*. We'd suggest you find a nutritionally oriented doctor and then walk calmly to him or her. For there's a lot of evidence that establishes a connection between diabetes (and diabetes-like symptoms) and vitamin C. But, before we discuss this connection, let's briefly talk about some of the disorder's characteristics.

Diabetes is fundamentally a metabolic disorder. In diabetes insipidus ("insipid" because volumes of dilute, almost watery fluid are urinated), the pituitary gland is functioning at half mast. In diabetes mellitus ("mellitus" being Latin for honey—meaning the sweetness of the sugar in one's urine), the pancreas is held to be at fault. Directly or indirectly, this fault is an insulin deficit. This result is *hyperglycemia*—too much sugar in the blood, which causes too much sugar in the urine, as well as urination that is too frequent and too voluminous. All this leaves a victim weak, thirsty, hungry, and subject to some profoundly serious upsets in body chemistry.

TEXTBOOKS VERSUS SCIENTIFIC JOURNALS

What do the experts tell us about a vitamin C connection in the control of sugar metabolism?

We turned to the ten leading textbooks dealing with diabetes mellitus published during the last decade. It's hard to believe, but we found not one word indicating any connection—or even a lack of connection!—between ascorbic acid and the metabolism of carbohydrates (the major sugar source).

Why is this hard to believe? It's hard to believe because some fascinating reports have been published in the medical literature over a period of roughly fifty years. Dice and Daniel of Stanford University comment on their own work: "The results of this pilot study suggest the need of well-controlled large scale tests to determine whether this observation [C's lowering blood-sugar glycemia] is true for other diabetics." Dr. Dice, who had been diagnosed as diabetic at age fifteen, served as his own guinea pig in this experiment. Unresponsive to then-popular pills for lowering blood sugar, he was taking insulin by injection. To test the C connection, he took progressively increasing amounts of ascorbic acid each hour from 7 A.M. to 1 A.M. When hypoglycemia (lowered blood sugar) occurred, he cut the daily amount of insulin. When glycosuria developed, he added more vitamin C. In this small study it was shown "that ascorbic acid exhibits marked hypoglycemic activity." We join Dice and Daniel in their hope that more work will be done with instances of juvenile-onset diabetes.

Fortunately, in the case of maturity-onset diabetes mellitus, the reports are more thorough, which only goes to deepen our wonderment that the research findings have not found their way into medical textbooks!

Early Work

As long ago as 1936, the *Journal of Biological Chemistry* featured a study by Sigal and King on vitamin C depletion in guinea pigs—those little creatures that, like humans, cannot synthesize their own. By means of glucose-tolerance tests, it was clearly demonstrated that progressive vitamin C depletion produces a state of chemical diabetes. In 1937, Pfleger and Scholl showed that C could reduce insulin requirements in insulin-dependent diabetics, without affecting glucose metabolism in diabetics not on insulin, or in "normals."

Just a few years later, Palle Hjorth of the Copenhagen Commune Hospital reviewed all the then-published scientific literature. He noted two important facts: (1) there was already a voluminous amount of information available pointing to a relationship between ascorbic acid and diabetes, and (2) confusion about interpreting the data probably resulted from varying techniques and the different kinds of patients (as well as presumably healthy people) studied.

With this frame of reference, Hjorth decided to find out whether administering vitamin C to individuals with low vitamin C blood-serum levels would cause any change in their glucose-tolerance patterns. Tests were performed at intervals of at least four days, then the subjects were given 200 to 500 mg of vitamin C intravenously every day for eight to ten days. After that, glucose-tolerance tests were repeated and before and after comparisons were made. The difference in curves indicated that "the carbohydrate assimilation improves when man is given an ample supply of ascorbic acid."

Still back in the 1940s, Ole Sylvest from the Old Age Pensioners' Town in Copenhagen conducted experiments in the morning hours under fasting conditions. After blood sugar and serum ascorbic-acid levels were taken, 0.5 to 1 gram of vitamin C was intravenously injected into patients. Then blood samples were obtained every twenty minutes over a three-hour period. While Sylvest claimed it is not possible to make any "rules" about the connection, he reported that a "lowering of the blood sugar has taken place in the majority of cases after intravenous injection of ascorbic acid."

At another Copenhagen setting, the Bispebjerg Hospital, Knud Secher reported that abnormally high blood-sugar levels of a diabetic type may be restored to more physiologic patterns by simply providing ascorbic-acid supplements to people with vitamin C deficiencies. Secher maintained that any decision regarding the significance of a blood-sugar picture is incomplete unless the blood's vitamin C content is also analyzed.

What a shame that even at this late date Dr. Secher's warning goes unheeded by "official" agencies entrusted with defining components of diabetes, as we'll see below.

More Recent Work

Just as is true today, the mid-1960s saw considerable controversy over what constitutes the "physiologic range" for vitamin C. The

Interdepartmental Committee on Nutrition for National Defense (ICNND) argued that plasma ascorbic-acid levels below 0.2 mg percent were unsatisfactory. Other observers regarded 0.5 mg percent as the cutoff point, while still others said the minimal level should be 0.6 mg percent or 0.7 mg percent.

We set about to study 169 randomly chosen and presumably healthy young adults, predominately female. Carbohydrate metabolism was rated by the then-popular cortisone glucose-tolerance test; plasma vitamin C levels were established under fasting conditions. Our objective was to see if there was significant parallelism between the two measurements in the largest experimental population ever used.

No matter how you slice the "C cutoff levels" noted above, a significant portion of these young and seemingly healthy people demonstrated below-optimal ascorbic-acid levels: if it's 0.2 mg percent, 30.2 percent; if it's 0.5 mg percent, 55 percent; if it's 0.6 mg percent, 61 percent; if it's 0.7 mg percent, 67.5 percent. In short, anywhere from 30 percent to almost 68 percent of our subjects were low on C.

Would being low on C match glucose tolerance? Both to sharpen the concept of "low" and also to provide large subgroups that could be meaningfully compared, we chose a cutoff point of 0.5 mg percent. This provided us with 103 subjects with plasma levels of 0.5 mg percent or less and 66 subjects with concentration of 0.6 mg percent or more.

At every measurement time, the lower–vitamin C group showed a more diabetic-like blood-sugar pattern. Also, in practically all instances, the "variances"—meaning the spread of values about the mean (arithmetic average)—in the two groups were distinctly and significantly different. What this says, in general, is that subjects with a relatively poor vitamin C state tend to have degrees of either hyperglycemia (high blood sugar) or hypoglycemia (low blood sugar).

We then asked: How will aging affect this picture?

We found the expected when average blood-glucose scores were higher in an older group of subjects *and* that the level peaked much later after a "glucose load" (high intake of sugar) than in younger subjects.

We also found the unexpected. In the older group with a low vitamin C state, there was a greater proneness to either hyper- or hypoglycemia. "Everyone" has long known that age is paralleled by a decrease in glucose tolerance; the question is whether this is "natural" (that is, a physiological part of aging) or whether it's pathological.

While our study confirms that glucose tolerance decreases with age, evidence we gathered shows that older people with healthy vitamin C pictures are not different from younger people in terms of blood-sugar levels. Generally speaking, the more C, the better the glucose tolerance.

It's handy to remember that what statisticians call "correlation" does *not* mean "cause and effect." For example, infant mortality increases and more ice-cream cones are consumed. The correlation or association: it's a hot summer. We're not saying there is a cause-and-effect relationship, but there is certainly an association—as our next study demonstrated.

This time our subjects were thirty-nine presumably healthy third-year dental students, most of them in their twenties. On Monday mornings, nonfasting (two hours *after* breakfast) blood glucose and plasma vitamin C were measured. Then the participants were randomly divided into an experimental group (twenty-three subjects) and a control group (fifteen subjects). Members of the first group reported each day at 7:45 A.M. and 1:30 P.M., at which time they swallowed 50 grams of sucrose in solution. On Friday of the same week, blood glucose and ascorbic-acid levels were remeasured by the same technician, who had no knowledge of the earlier findings or whether subjects were in the sucrose or the nonsucrose group.

The average change in blood sugar in the control group was quite insignificant (less than 1 percent). But in the subjects who had received the sugar solutions there was an average decline of 13 percent. This average, while significant in itself, was just the average. Some subjects showed a greater decrease, others less. When we compared their ratings against vitamin C states—with 0.7 mg percent as the cutoff point—we found that the less blood-glucose fluctuation, the better the subject's C state.

SOME TENTATIVE CONCLUSIONS

Clearly there is a vitamin C connection in diabetes, even though descriptions of the syndrome as "liberal" as that of S. S. Fajans do not spell it out word for word, and even though reports by the American Diabetes Association fail to mention it at all.

But contemporary research is echoing findings made forty and nearly fifty years ago, and it's not just in terms of sugar metabolism but also involves energy metabolism as a whole and the relationship of vitamin C to many other body substances and functions.

For example, the Czech researcher Emil Ginter—by now an old friend to readers of this book—sought to clarify C's connection to serum cholesterol in diabetic subjects. His conclusion? "A significantly lower vitamin C concentration has been found in the blood and particularly in the leukocytes of hypercholesterolemic [too much blood cholesterol] diabetic patients than of healthy blood donors. Ascorbic acid administered in a dose of 500 mg per day for 12 months to metabolically stabilize hypercholesterolemic subjects with maturity-onset diabetes mellitus brought about a striking decline of cholesterolemia and a moderate decline of triglyceridemia. The serum lipid level in the control group remained unaltered. *These data underline the necessity of monitoring vitamin C status in diabetic patients and in case the values are low, to increase the intake of vitamin C* [italics added]."

We need to know more, but we know enough to urge diabetics and others with hyper- or hypoglycemic problems to consult a nutritionally oriented doctor who understands the vitamin C connection.

10

The Two C's in Cancer

Our title is not a word game. It refers to two ways vitamin C can combat the dreaded disease of cancer: (1) through therapeutic actions, it may keep victims alive; and (2) by enhancing immune mechanisms, it may prevent a person from "getting" the disease in the first place.

SOME FRIGHTENING FIGURES

About one in four Americans now living—that is, approximately 56 million people—will eventually have cancer. This means some two out of every three families will be affected.

The decade of the 1970s saw an incidence increase of between 5 and 10 percent. In the last four years of the 1970s, annual cancer deaths rose from 377,312 to 386,686 to 392,000 to about 399,000.

Currently, scientists are able to predict that, each year, about 785,000 people will be diagnosed as having cancer. (This estimate omits some 400,000 people who will be found to have skin cancer of a nonmelanoma type.) Approximately 405,000 people died of this disease during 1980. This comes to 1100 people daily—that is, a death every 78 seconds.

Cancer does more than kill. It causes enormous psychological stress—often more to family and friends than to the victim. It imposes terrible financial burdens, costing, on the average, more than $20,000 for direct medical services. According to a Department of Health, Education, and Welfare report, fiscal year

1975—still the most recent year for which figures are available—showed $5.3 billion as the direct cost for treating neoplasms (abnormal growths that are mostly cancers). The economic hardships extend also to lost earning power estimated at between $13.7 and $22.7 billion annually.

SOME QUICK QUESTIONS

"Will I be the one in four?" "Will someone in my family be stricken?" "Is there anything I can *do?*"

Our answer to the third question hinges on the vitamin C connections outlined in this chapter. Your answers to the following questions may suggest your own susceptibility, or that of a loved one. We are talking about *potential* only. But the more YES answers you circle, the more apt you are to take a personalized interest in the research findings we're about to describe. First, the test:

Is there a history of cancer in your family?	YES	NO
Do you smoke?	YES	NO
Is one of these foods in your diet almost every day— bacon, hot dogs, luncheon meats, sliced sandwich meats, ham, corned beef?	YES	NO
Do you usually avoid citrus fruit and juices?	YES	NO
Are you susceptible to colds and other infections?	YES	NO
Do you frequently consume sweetened foods and beverages?	YES	NO
Do you drink some kind of alcoholic beverage daily?	YES	NO
Do you usually avoid taking vitamin supplements?	YES	NO
Do you frequently take an over-the-counter sedative?	YES	NO
Have you ever had a cancer or tumor?	YES	NO
Do you often go through a day without having a bowel movement?	YES	NO
Do you have diabetes or hypoglycemia?	YES	NO
So far, have you made lots of positive responses to the questions that open most chapters of this book?	YES	NO

SOME REASONABLE REMINDERS

The Body's Defense Lines

In Chapter 3 we outlined how the body's immune system works. This complex set of biologic and chemical processes involves cell-mediated and humoral immunity. This includes antibody production, the formation and activity of lymphocytes, as well as the attraction to and destruction of microbes known as neutrophilic chemotaxis and phagocytosis, respectively. The reader who wants a better understanding of how some of these processes work may wish to turn back to "How Not to Be Bugged by Infection" for another runthrough on the subject. The important things to keep in mind, however, are that the body has coping mechanisms against foreign and "mutant" invaders—including cancer—and that vitamin C is essential for these mechanisms to operate successfully.

In the context of cancer, you might find it useful to picture the immune system as a police force that constantly patrols the body, keeping an eye open for cells that are becoming neoplastic—that is, growing in unexpected (and usually dangerous) ways. Vitamin C not only stimulates this immune system, both before and after a diagnosis of cancer, but it also has been shown to kill cancer cells themselves.

JUST WHAT *IS* CANCER?

The word neoplasm means, quite literally, "new growth." In cancer, this "new growth" occurs when cells go berserk—frequently forming a malignant tumor and often spreading or *metastasizing* to other parts of the body. You may hear of several types. In *carcinoma,* epithelium, the membrane that covers external and internal body surfaces, including cavities and the lining of vessels, infiltrates other tissues and often metastasizes. *Sarcomas,* cancers of connective tissues and bone, feature an embryoniclike tissue gone haywire. *Melanomas* of the malignant type may start out with a circumscribed center (maybe a dark-colored mole) and then spread their black cell masses out and about. Of course, there are many more subgroupings and individually named cancers—like Hodgkin's disease or "pseudoleukemia"; "real" leukemia, which affects lymph tissue and blood-forming organs, causing an enormous increase in leukocytes; those associated with certain occupations; and many others.

No matter what the type or the special name, each malignant tumor shares this common pathology: cells run amuck and grow in unnatural, life-threatening ways. No one is quite sure exactly why and how this happens. But we do know that there is a definite vitamin C connection that deserves at least as much attention as the toxic drugs that are approved for anticancer use. We hope that the various research studies described below will stimulate further interest in *non*toxic approaches to the prevention and treatment of cancer.

THE FIRST C: PREVENTION

The measurement scale may have changed, but the sentiment is the same: "28 grams of prevention is worth 0.45 kilograms of cure."

On July 15, 1980, an Associated Press release from Washington, D.C., stated that "some chemicals may protect people against cancer" and that, from animal test data, "such chemicals as vitamins A and C may stave off cancer under certain circumstances."

These words came from Vincent T. DeVita, the then-new head of the National Cancer Institute. Dr. DeVita also commented that "the Cancer Institute is giving greater attention to cancer prevention."

How *much* attention still remains to be seen. Meanwhile, back in the laboratories and clinical settings, researchers continue to strengthen the vitamin C connection.

The abnormal-behaving cells characteristic of the diseases we call "cancer" are constantly being generated in our bodies. What keeps us from "getting" the disease is the wide array of tumor-cell destroyers that cruise about our body. Griffiths and co-workers have shown that about 50 percent of patients about to undergo surgery for cancer of the colon or rectum have malignant cells circulating about the body through the blood stream. However, many of these patients survive, seemingly well and cured, for many years. Since there was no cancer recurrence, it's obvious that these circulating malignant cells were somehow destroyed.

How?

The patients' immune mechanisms—just like ours—may succeed in their search-and-destroy mission. These defenders are largely dependent on vitamin C, in ways described in Chapter 3. Ascorbic acid seems also to combat malignancy directly. For example, two researchers at Children's Hospital in Los Angeles, William F. Benedict and Peter A. Jones, examined ascorbic acid's effect on mouse-embryo cells exposed to carcinogenic (cancer-causing) agents. Cell transformation was completely blocked for as long as twenty-three days. Even after cells had altered to a tumor-suggesting state, vitamin C caused 75 percent of them to revert to normal.

For some twenty years Sister Mary Eymard Poydock, Ph.D. (Professor of Biology and Director of Cancer Research at Mercyhurst College in Erie, Pennsylvania), worked with associates at Saint Thomas' Institute in Cincinnati in a series of in vivo and in vitro lower-animal experiments. They found that a combination of vitamin C and vitamin B_{12}, which they dubbed Mercytamin, definitely inhibits mitosis or division of neoplastic cells—without affecting normal ones. Higher doses of vitamin C alone also showed some capability of curbing the division of cancer cells. These researchers reported that the C-B_{12} combination is effective against sarcomas, carcinomas, and leukemias.

How about *people?* A University of Kansas Medical Center group headed by Chan H. Park showed that vitamin C can suppress the growth of leukemic cells from human beings. When weak concentrations (0.1 to 0.3 mM) of ascorbic acid were added to the culture medium, the number of leukemic cell colonies was reduced by 21 percent. No damage was done to normal myeloid precursor cells (types of "baby cells" in bone marrow).

Some French scientists and Stanley Bram's group at Baylor University School of Medicine demonstrated that vitamin C is toxic to malignant melanoma cells from humans. The addition of tissue saturation concentrations (1 to 2 mM) of vitamin C to the cell culture resulted in a 50 percent decrease in colony formation.

And not all the work has been done in vitro (in the test tube). Robert Yonemoto, a surgeon and Director of Surgical Laboratories at City of Hope National Medical Center in Duarte, California, along with two colleagues from the National Cancer Institute (Chretien and Fehniger) worked with healthy young adults. The subjects were given 5 grams of ascorbic acid daily for three days. In response to the "challenge" of an immune-system stimulant, lymphocyte blastogenesis—a cell division resulting in the rapid multiplication of a type of cancer-combating white blood cell—increased significantly. The increase was even greater when 10 grams of vitamin C was given daily for three days.

These researchers say that lymphocyte blastogenesis becomes more and more impaired with advancing cancer, and the state of this mechanism should correlate well with a patient's prognosis. In a seemingly healthy person, impaired blastogenesis from vitamin C deprivation could also warn of susceptibility to cancer.

Jorgen V. Schlegel and associates at Tulane University's School of Medicine are among the groups of researchers who have shown that substances found in human urine may cause cancer of the urinary bladder. Some of these naturally occurring substances are metabolites of the dietary amino acid called L-tryptophan, and most of them are carcinogenic in experimental animals. Researchers believe that the oxygen-scavenging action of vitamin C can block the substances from reacting with oxygen in the bladder so that they are not transformed into carcinogens. After first working with mice, Dr. Schlegel now routinely administers 1000 to 1500 mg of C daily to patients who have bladder tumors and are in a high-risk category from smoking or drinking large amounts of alcohol, cola, or coffee. The aim is to exceed the body's requirements so that vitamin C spills into the urine. Once this state is maintained, no new bladder cancers develop—as was confirmed in the report by Schlegel and Pipkin.

Vitamin C may also offer new hope for the distressingly high number of women stricken by cancer of the cervix. A team from the Johns Hopkins University School of Hygiene and Public Health, headed by Sylvia Wassertheil-Smoller, reported on a research project that involved 169 participants. Of these women, 87 had cervical dysplasias (abnormalities) detected by Pap smears; 82 "normals" served as controls. The role of vitamin C was separated out from other variables (such as age and sexual activity) and matched-pairs analysis showed results that are summarized below.

	CONTROLS	POSITIVES	LEVEL OF STATISTICAL SIGNIFICANCE
Average daily C intake	107 mg	80 mg	<0.01
Proportion with less than half the RDA	3%	29%	<0.05

As you can see, below-RDA levels of vitamin C intake mean a *tenfold* increase in the risk of cervical dysplasia.

Since about "35% of US women in their reproductive years have daily vitamin C intake below 30 mg, and 68% have vitamin C intake below 88 mg," the researchers conclude that it should be valuable "to explore a possible protective role of supplementary vitamin C for women at high risk of cervical cancer."

The Nitrite Scene

Of course, "internal" chemicals are not the only ones people must contend with. Foods, tobacco smoke, flavoring agents, pesticides, herbicides, and a variety of therapeutic drugs contain amines. Like amides, a urea, or a urethane, amines can combine with a nitrite (nitrosation) before or after it hits the stomach. This combination forms an N-nitroso compound—sometimes called a *nitrosamine*—that can cause cancer in lower animals. Since no species is known to be resistant to these chemicals, there is good reason to believe humans are susceptible, as is contended by William Lijinsky (Eppley Institute for Research in Cancer, University of Nebraska College of Medicine) and Samuel Epstein (Children's Cancer Research Foundation and Department of Pathology, Harvard Medical School).

It's hard to avoid these substances if you eat! Nitrate, which is converted to nitrite by a variety of microorganisms, is an important component of crop fertilizers. Sodium nitrite is used in meat processing to suppress bacterial growth (especially the botulinum bacteria) and to lend some color and flavor to cured meat products. Some commonly eaten vegetables from treated crops can contain up to 4031 ppm (parts per million) of nitrate, which can cause an alarmingly high concentration of salivary nitrite. Tannenbaum and co-workers feel this should wield "a major influence on thinking concerning the health effects of nitrate in the environment."

This concern is echoed by a group of researchers at the Roche Research Center in Nutley, New Jersey, who say that it is "of considerable importance to eliminate or significantly reduce the potential threat to human health imposed by man's ingestion of nitrite and amines or preformed nitrosamines," and by N. Lee Wolfe and Richard Zepp of the Environmental Protection Agency's laboratory at Athens, Georgia. Wolfe and Zepp report that atrazine, a widely used pesticide, will react with nitrite under acidic conditions to form a nitrosamine. This situation is of immediate concern because atrazine residues have already been found in drinking water in Iowa and Louisiana.

Finally, "bringing home the bacon" may no longer be a laudable goal. When nitrite-cured bacon is cooked, the nitrite changes to nitrous acid, which then reacts with amines in the meat to form dimethyl nitrosamine, a potential carcinogen. Other nitrite-containing American favorites? Hot dogs, luncheon meats, sliced sandwich meats, ham, and corned beef. Perhaps Homoganized Bakon—a nitrite-free precooked bacon patented by R. A. Kennedy and approved by the United States Department of Agriculture—will blaze a path for other companies to follow in minimizing nitrosamine hazards in our environment.

In the meantime, how does vitamin C fit in? It has been shown to effectively prevent nitrosamine formation in a number of food products, such as hot dogs, bacon, and potatoes. When boiled potatoes were incubated in an acid environment simulating the stomach, the more ascorbic acid was added, the less methylnitrosourea was formed. Findings reported by Weisburger and team are summarized below.

Effect of Ascorbic Acid on the Formation of Methylnitrosourea in Potatoes Incubated at pH 1.5

METHYLUREA	NITRITE	ASCORBATE : NITRITE RATIO	METHYLNITROSOUREA FORMED (PPM)	INHIBITION (%)
100 ppm	100 ppm	0	19.0	0
100 ppm	100 ppm	1	12.0	37
100 ppm	100 ppm	2	5.0	74
100 ppm	100 ppm	4	1.4	93

Various research studies have demonstrated how vitamin C alters chemical reactions so that nitrites can't combine with available amines or other substances to form toxic nitroso compounds. Among published reports are studies (in vitro and in vivo) by Mirvish and his associates at the Eppley Institute for Research in Cancer (University of Nebraska Medical Center); a group headed by L. Lakritz of the Eastern Region Research Center in Philadelphia (working with nineteen males and nineteen females); William R. Bruce and co-workers at the Ontario Cancer Institute in Toronto (cancer patients and "normals"); and John H. Weisburger of the American Health Foundation in Valhalla, New York.

A number of drugs may also potentiate nitroso activity in the stomach. We suggest you check your medicine cabinet or ask your pharmacist or doctor to find out whether you or a family member is taking any drug whose generic name is piperazine, phenmetrazine, primaquine, pamaquine, physostigmine, synephrine, sulfanilylurea, neohydrin, oxytetracycline, or morpholine. Dr. Sidney Mirvish and his team at the Eppley Institute for Research in Cancer say that the nitroso hazard "might be reduced by administering the drug together with a substance that preferentially reacts with and destroys any nitrite occurring in the stomach." They add that "vitamin C might be used for this purpose."

This advice can probably be applied to the swallowing of many different kinds of pills. G. S. Rao, a researcher for the American Dental Association in Chicago, says that twenty amine-containing prescription drugs will react with sodium nitrite in the stomach to form several nitroso compounds—about half of which are known carcinogens. Many nonprescription sedatives used to contain methapyrilene, which reacted with stomach nitrites to form one of the most potent carcinogens known: dimethylnitrosamine. Until recently methapyrilene was found in a number of over-the-counter sedatives.

How We See C

Cancer specialists know there is a good correlation between how chemotherapy drugs act on freshly obtained malignant cells from a cancer patient and how the patient will clinically respond to the same drugs. We know that vitamin C suppresses leukemic cells in test-tube (in vitro) experiments. In vivo work (studies with people) can be easily and safely done because the equivalent of the C dosage used in vitro can be readily achieved with a pharmacologic dose of L-ascorbic acid. The same goes for melanoma, in which the Bram group worked in vitro.

We've mentioned in this chapter and outlined in more detail in Chapter 3 how vitamin C activates the immune system. Another important anticancer influence comes from ascorbic acid's stimulating production of the cellular substance called adenosine 3, 5-monophosphate or 3, 5-cyclic AMP or, simply, cyclic AMP. In cell culture fluid, cyclic AMP has inhibited cancer-cell proliferation from 70 to 89 percent, with only a slight effect on nonmalignant cells. And, in a cell culture of fibroblasts, cyclic AMP produced a significant increase in the antiviral activity of interferon—which could be an important mechanism for inhibiting virus-induced cancers. We'd like to see more work done in these areas.

Ewan Cameron (Vale of Leven Hospital, Scotland) and Nobel laureate Linus Pauling maintain that cancer cells are restrained from expanding by a chemical known as physiologic hyaluronidase inhibitor, or PHI. They explain that *all* tissue cells tend to divide, but are restrained by the gluey intercellular substances called glycosamino-glycans, which are dense because of their high molecular weights. Hyaluronidase alters this glue around cells and permits them to wander. This will continue as long as the chemical is released but "proliferation will cease and normal tissue restraint and organization will be restored when the production of hyaluronidase returns to normal."

Hyaluronidase inhibitor (PHI) contains ascorbic acid in its molecular structure and it requires C for synthesis. Cameron and Pauling feel "there is accumulating evidence that ascorbic acid is involved in a whole pattern of specific biochemical reactions that collectively enhance host resistance to malignant invasive growth." In cancer, cells "in becoming malignant have acquired, and are able to bequeath to their descendants *in perpetuo,* the ability to produce hyaluronidase continually."

Vitamin C supplementation certainly seems to make sense! It's been reported that 88 percent of all cancers originate from organs that contain less than 4.5 mg of vitamin C per 100 grams of organ tissue. Only 12 percent of cancers originate from organs containing higher concentrations.

THE SECOND C: TREATMENT

Cancer does not end the *preventive* roles played by vitamin C. That is, immune reactions and other defense mechanisms are still enhanced by ascorbic acid even in cancer patients. But now we turn to the second C: Can vitamin C directly stop the growth and/or spread of cancer?

One of the first published reports about using vitamin C to treat cancer patients came in 1954 from Dr. Edward Greer of Illinois. The patient, a seventy-year-old executive for an oil company, was suffering from chronic myelogenous leukemia—plus cirrhosis of the liver, arthritis, a blood disorder marked by too many red cells, and a heart problem. On Dr. Greer's two-year, 20- to 40-gram daily vitamin C regimen, the man repeatedly remarked about his general feeling of well-being and continued to work. Whenever—as part of the "experiment"—he discontinued the C, his spleen enlarged, his temperature rose to 101° F, and he reported fatigue and general malaise. His liver and spleen also became enlarged as well as soft and tender. When he resumed taking vitamin C, these signs and symptoms subsided.

Of course, this is but one case report. However, there are many others. In Chapter 21 of his book *Vitamin C and Cancer*, Linus Pauling cites twenty-six case histories which indicate "that supplemental ascorbate is of some value in all forms of cancer and can prove to be of dramatic benefit to a fortunate few." Along with Campbell and Jack, Cameron reports complete remission in a forty-two-year-old carcinoma victim given 10 grams of ascorbic acid each day.

Nor has the research been confined to single-case reports. At the University of Glasgow and the University Hospital of South Manchester, Krasner and Dymock worked with fifty patients suffering from metastatic cancer, spread from primary sites such as the bronchus, stomach, colon, rectum, pancreas, brain, prostate, liver, breast, and reticular system. They found that forty-six of these patients had white-blood-cell vitamin C levels below the lower limit of normal, with thirty of them having extremely subnormal levels. The latter exhibited signs and symptoms of low-grade scurvy—hemorrhages under the tongue, decreased capillary strength, and skin and hair abnormalities. The investigators concluded that most cancer patients have minimal stores of vitamin C and should be receiving supplements.

At Vale of Leven Hospital in Loch Lomondside, Cameron and Pauling administered 10 grams of sodium ascorbate daily to fifty terminal cancer patients expected to die within ninety days. The remarkable result? They proved not so terminal—in the *immediate* sense of the term—when given vitamin C. Although half of them did die on or before Day 100, twenty survived as long as 659 days (average, 261 days), and five were still living when the report was written. Furthermore, all the patients showed general clinical improvement, indicating a lessening of malignant activity, along with relief from pain.

In another treatment trial at the same hospital, one hundred terminal cancer patients given 10 grams of sodium ascorbate each day were compared with one thousand patients who were not given this supplement. As Cameron and Pauling report, the survival ratio for C subjects proved to be 4.2, 5.6, and 6.6 greater than for the controls—according to the times at which comparisons were made. At last report, five patients were still living and taking their daily dose of sodium ascorbate. It is said that "some of them might well be considered to have been 'cured' of their malignant disease, in that they are free of overt manifestations of cancer and are leading normal lives."

Cameron and Pauling, as well as many other scientists, are optimistic about future application of all these clinical findings. Lest a reader ascribe this optimism to the enthusiasm of *people,* let us turn to the cold eye of statistical analysis. Professor George A. Farrah of the Center for Educational Administration and Leadership at St. Cloud University in Minnesota, where he is also Director of Field Studies, decided to take a good look at the data from Vale of Leven. Employing a highly sophisticated variance/covariance model of his own design, Professor Farrah first concluded that the level of statistical significance in survival time was even greater than claimed by Cameron and Pauling. Farrah sets the level-of-confidence at 97.4 percent for twelve of the types of cancer and 99.5 percent for six of them. What this means is there are only a few chances in ten thousand that the better results reflect some accidental occurrence!

While Edward T. Creagan and his associates at the Mayo Clinic in Rochester, Minnesota, failed to duplicate the Vale of Leven findings, it should be noted that 87 percent of their ascorbate-treated patients had received prior courses of chemotherapy. Only 4 percent of the Vale of Leven subjects had. Since cytotoxic (cell-poisoning) chemotherapy damages the immune system, it can cancel vitamin C's effect and block the anticancer attack.

In Japan, a five-year study by Morishige and Murata brought results more in line with the Vale of Leven findings. Working with ninty-nine patients classified as terminally ill with cancer, Morishige and Murata administered varying amounts of ascorbic acid—forty-four received 4 grams or less each day (average, 1.5) and fifty-five received 5 grams or more daily (average, 29).

More than five years after the project was started, six "terminal" patients were still living. Each of them had been in the higher-dose category—but, interestingly, three of them had been receiving "as little" as 6 grams (6000 mg) per day. The overall average survival time for 33 percent of the higher-dose group was 483 days. Not a single member of the lower-dose group lived longer than 174 days. Doctors Morishige and Murata conclude: "Supplemental vitamin C in large doses has significant benefit for patients with advanced cancer."

A group from the Ontario Cancer Treatment and Research Foundation and Western Reserve University, headed by C. J. Koch, discovered that vitamin C is a valuable addition to the treatment of radiation-resistant tumor cells. When ascorbic acid is added to nitroaromatic radiosensitizing drugs, the latter's toxicity is greatly increased so that "sick cells" can be killed.

Another team, from the Vince Lombardi Colon Clinic in Milwaukee, headed by Jerome J. DeCosse, chose to work with *pre*-malignant patients. Colonic polyposis is a genetic disease characterized by many polyps in the colon and rectum; it is widely thought to be a precursor to cancer. Administration of 3 grams (3000 mg) daily of ascorbic acid caused improvement ranging from a 35 percent lessening of polyp density to complete disappearance of the growths. Pathologist Basil C. Morson of St. Mark's Hospital in London is currently running a double-blind study to check Dr. DeCosse's results.

LIFE AND THREE ORANGES

What's the Next Step?

In an opera fairy tale, a prince finds love through three oranges. Can our "average American" Polly or Paul find *life* through vitamin C? Research shows how ascorbic acid acts against cancer, but not all scientists agree; could they believe it's only a fairy tale?

Here's what Dr. Samuel Klein had to say after conducting an exhaustive review of the medical/scientific literature:

> History has demonstrated the resistance of scientists to unorthodox ideas. Mendel's theories on inheritance, Pasteur's germ theory and Semmelweis' desire for antiseptic procedures were rejected by the sci-

entific communities of their times. Cancer, a disease of great psychological impact, is a vulnerable target for unorthodox methods of treatment. It is too easy, however, to categorize all agents as quackery, and one must separate emotional bias from scientific fact. *There are many areas where ascorbic acid may play a significant role in the prevention or treatment of human cancers.* Full research is needed to ascertain its full potential. [italics added]

We think Dr. Klein is right. And we'd be the first to applaud massive research that could reveal vitamin C's *full* potential in this connection. At the same time, we see no logical reason why the clinical use of ascorbic acid should be withheld while we all wait for more research results that confirm what everyone knows already.

"What everyone knows already" amounts to the following: many studies have shown that vitamin C has a definite effect on the prevention and the treatment of cancer; vitamin C is relatively nontoxic and "absolutely nontoxic" when compared with the many highly toxic chemotherapeutic drugs in current use. We find it interesting, but sad, that sublethal amounts of toxic drugs are approved for use with a minimum quantity of preliminary evidence, but nutritional therapies are expected to wait for some sort of "final proof of effectiveness" before they can swim down the mainstream of medical practice.

Surely it behooves people with cancer, or who come from cancer-prone families, to seek out a nutritionally oriented doctor for direction and supervision of vitamin C administration.

11
The "Tired Blood" Caper

"Tired blood" is one of the more felicitous phrases brought to us by Madison Avenue. On our TV screens we see its agonized victims listlessly wandering about the house or their favorite pharmacy in search of Femiron, Mol-Iron, or that venerable product for "venerable" people (over age thirty-five!), Geritol.

Are you dogged by the symptoms of tired blood? You can grade your tiredness by counting YES answers to a few questions adapted from the Cornell Medical Index Health Questionnaire (CMI).

Do you often get spells of complete exhaustion or fatigue?	YES	NO
Does working tire you out completely?	YES	NO
Do you usually get up tired and exhausted in the morning?	YES	NO
Does every little effort wear you out?	YES	NO
Are you constantly too tired and exhausted even to eat?	YES	NO
Do you suffer from severe "nervous exhaustion"?	YES	NO
Does "nervous exhaustion" run in your family?	YES	NO

If you think you have "tired blood," you might want to consider supplementing iron intake with vitamin C. It plays a role in iron absorption, and a lack of ascorbic acid can cause profound degrees of fatigue and exhaustion from an iron deficit. However, before we discuss vitamin C's connection to "tired blood," let's check out anemia and iron intake.

FERROUS FADING

Iron—*ferrum* to the Latin student and simply Fe to the chemistry student—is essential to "healthy blood." It's especially vital to hemoglobin, that oxygen-carrying pigment of red blood cells. Vital it may be, but G. H. Beaton (Department of Nutrition at the School of Hygiene, Toronto University) reminds us that it is generally believed "that in industrial countries iron deficiency is the most widespread form of nutritional deficiency" and that refined techniques have opened up new avenues for epidemiologic investigation.

The Committee on Dietary Allowances of the Food and Nutrition Board covers an enormous portion of the population with the statement that follows:

> There are four situations in which iron intake is frequently inadequate in the United States: (1) in infancy, because of the low iron content of milk and because the endowment of iron at birth is usually not sufficient to meet needs beyond six months; (2) during the periods of rapid growth in childhood and adolescence, because of the need to fill expanding iron stores; (3) during the female reproductive period, because of menstrual iron losses; and (4) in pregnancy, because of the expanding blood volume of the mother, the demands of the fetus and placenta, and blood losses in childbirth.

In a study of 370 low-income adolescents in the South, Elaine G. Gaines and W. A. Daniel at the University of Alabama in Birmingham Medical Center found that "the majority of the subjects consumed less than the recommended allowances of iron." Moving up in age to adults, James D. Cox and his colleagues in the Division of Hematology at the University of Washington in Seattle studied the iron status of 1564 subjects living in the Northwest. Three indices—transferrin saturation, red cell protoporphyrin, and serum ferritin—were used. When one of the three was studied, 10.9 percent showed abnormality; with two, 28 percent; with all three, 63 percent. This underscores a well-known saying in diagnostics: "The harder one looks, the more one finds." It also shows an almost epidemic incidence of iron deficiency.

In a population of people in late middle age, Mary Bess Kohrs and associates found "a significant proportion of the men [20 percent] and women [10 percent] had low hemoglobin levels" as well as low levels of serum iron. This rate was upped to an overall total of 40 percent when elderly institutionalized patients were studied over a one-year period by Thomas Kalchthaler and M. Eunice Rigor Tan at Saint Joseph's Hospital Nursing Home in Yonkers, New York.

The same governmental committee quoted earlier in this book says that adult males and postmenopausal women need 10 mg of iron each day to retain the 1 mg needed. The allowance for women of childbearing age is set at 18 mg per day to offset menstrual losses. Noting that the "increased requirement during pregnancy cannot be met by the iron content of habitual diets in the United States," the experts recommend that pregnant women take daily supplements of iron, ranging from 30 to 60 mg daily.

Is It the Iron?

There are many reasons for "exhaustion." Certainly iron-deficiency anemia is among them, and we have no intention of downgrading iron's importance. But in the professional and public thrust to attach a lack of iron to "tired blood," very little attention has been directed to the possibility of a vitamin C connection—even though Dr. James Lind made note of such a relationship way back in 1753.

VITAMIN C AND FATIGUE

Our tireless Scots surgeon from the eighteenth century wrote a description that might serve an actress or actor in any "tired-blood" commercial. "The first indication of the approach of this

disease [scurvy] is generally a change in colour in the face, from
the natural and usual look, to a pale and bloated complexion; with
a listlessness to action, or an aversion to any sort of exercise. . . .
Meanwhile, the person eats and drinks heartily, and seems in perfect health; except that his countenance and lazy inactive disposition, portend a future scurvy."

Miniscurvy

One of the reasons there are fewer vitamin C connection reports
in the scientific literature, as compared with other diseases we've
discussed, is that full-blown, classical scurvy is relatively rare. The
scientific community seems not to hunt for *shades* of the disease.
But is this an all-or-none proposition? Might it not be possible to
suffer with, let us say, 50 percent scurvy? Common sense suggests
that, just as there are shades of gray, anger, obesity, and just
about everything else, there must be gradations of C deficiency.
And, since most people have trouble recognizing a thing for
which there is no name, let's call the disorder subclinical scurvy,
hemiscurvy, or semiscurvy, or demiscurvy, or—perhaps most
popularly—miniscurvy.

E. V. Cox contends there is a definite connection between C
and anemia; he reports that 80 percent of scorbutics are anemic.
This means that "tired blood" need not reflect a lack of iron. It
could entail vitamin C deficiency, or perhaps a combination of
the two factors.

We set about to compare tiredness with vitamin C consumption. For the former, we used fatigability signs and symptoms
from the Cornell questionnaire; for the latter, reported daily C
intake. Among our 411 subjects (dentists and their spouses),
eighty-one were taking less than 100 mg of vitamin C each day;
their average fatigability score was 0.81. The three-hundred individuals who were taking more than 400 mg of C per day (almost
seven times the so-called RDA) averaged a tiredness score of only
0.41—just about twice the resistance to fatigue or exhaustion.

As we've taken pains to point out elsewhere in this book, a
relationship or degree of correlation does not necessarily imply a

cause-and-effect chain. But there seems to be a parallelism that should interest other researchers—not to mention individuals suffering from "tired blood."

Iron Metabolism

It's been known for a long time that different types of iron, such as ferric versus ferrous compounds, are absorbed differently.

In the search for substances that can enhance iron absorption, one factor that keeps cropping up is vitamin C.

At research facilities in Göteborg, Sweden, Hans Brise and Leif Hallberg employed two radioiron isotopes in an experiment in which each subject could serve as his or her own control. They concluded that "orally administered ascorbic acid in sufficient amounts increases the absorption of iron from ferrous sulphate." They found that intravenous administration did not have this effect, so they believe that the vitamin C works because of "its reducing action within the gastrointestinal lumen, preventing or delaying a formation of insoluble or less dissociated ferric compounds."

Miguel Layrisse and co-workers at the Instituto Venzolano de Investigaciones Cientificas in Venezuela compared the effects of various kinds of animal foods and fruits on iron absorption. Most foods did not "work," although beef and fish muscle had some effect. But the most striking absorption came when papaya with high vitamin C content was used. Similar results were obtained by Sayers and associates at the University of Witwatersrand in Johannesburg, South Africa. Working with ascorbic acid added to various kinds of foods, they reported that—as we noted in the chapter called "Vitamin C's Vanishing Act"—such supplementation can prevent cooking or baking from ruining ascorbic acid's effects.

Fortifying the Defense Lines Since vitamin C is so unstable and iron seems to be in such short supply in most diets, wouldn't it be desirable to supply them on a mass basis—like fluoridating water supplies?

The South African group mentioned above chose to fortify salt with iron and vitamin C. Salt was used as a carrier for both iron and vitamin C added to rice-containing meals. The result: a threefold increase in iron uptake. This led Sayers and his colleagues to conclude that "the nutrition of rice-eating communities could be improved significantly by the addition of ascorbic acid to the diet." A slight hitch arose from the standpoint of esthetics: the salt looked dirty and discolored; a dab of starch took care of that. The researchers drew further pro-fortification conclusions about populations for whom maize forms a staple food.

A team headed by Lena Rossander at the Department of Medicine at the University of Göteborg (Sweden) conducted a series of nine experiments in which fortification was tested on a total of 129 presumably healthy people (65 men and 64 women) between the ages of seventeen and forty-six. Their report is published in the *American Journal of Clinical Nutrition*. Scientific-minded readers may want to consult it for all the minute details of exactly how everything was cooked and what the subjects' breakfasts consisted of, once the two subgroups were first given two different radioiron isotopes.

In essence, results can be summarized by a quotation from the researchers' report: "Adding orange juice to the basal breakfast more than doubled the iron absorption . . . if tea were served instead of coffee with the basal breakfast meal, the [iron] absorption decreased . . . the negative effect of tea could be counteracted by simultaneously serving orange juice."

We are reminded that it is availability, not basic content, that counts. "The main finding in this study reaffirms that dietary iron has to be evaluated according to its availability from food rather than simply by the iron content of food. Clearly, there is a marked effect of the composition of the breakfast meal on the absorption. Tea and orange juice have the greatest negative and positive effects [respectively]."

James D. Cook and Elaine R. Monsen, from the Division of Hematology at the University of Washington in Seattle, also used radioiron absorption tests to ascertain the effect C has on iron absorption. In sixty-three presumably healthy men ranging in age from eighteen to thirty-two, iron absorption from a semi-synthetic meal was directly proportional to the amount of vitamin C added—from a low of 25 to a high of 1000 mg. The 1.65 to 9.57 respective figures (ratio of iron absorption with and without ascorbic acid) show a difference that is nearly sixfold. An additional, and noteworthy, finding was that vitamin C taken only in the morning does *not* influence iron absorption from later meals. The hint? Spread your ascorbic-acid intake throughout the day. This hint draws further support from other University of Washington studies, all of which demonstrated a very good rate (about fivefold) of increased iron absorption when subjects were taking supplemental C.

The way vitamin C aids iron absorption is illustrated in the table that follows. Starting with a baseline absorption of 1 mg a day, the level increases according to the amount of ascorbic acid taken. You can also see that when the C is taken in divided doses during the day iron absorption increases even more dramatically—up to more than double the single-dose effect with breakfast.

Estimated Effect of Vitamin C Supplement on Iron Balance

DAILY SUPPLEMENTAL VITAMIN C (MG)	DAILY IRON ABSORPTION (MG)	
	WITH BREAKFAST	THREE DIVIDED DOSES
0	1.0	1.0
50–100	1.4	1.8
250–350	1.9	3.4
500	2.2	4.2
750	2.4	5.0
1000	2.7	5.7
2000	3.3	7.7
280*	1.9	3.3

*Average amount taken by subjects in the Cook and Monsen study.

The Heme Factor   Heme iron, present in the cells of animals, is an iron constituent of hemoglobin. It accounts for 40 percent of animal-tissue iron. The Food and Nutrition Board says that the other 60 percent, nonheme iron, from animal tissues and *all* iron in vegetable products, is "enhanced by two well-defined factors . . . ascorbic acid and the quantity of animal tissues present in each meal. On the basis of the concentration of these two enhancing factors, meals can be classified as of low, medium or high availability of their nonheme iron."

Examples: Low, Medium, High Iron

| | CONTENT | IRON ABSORPTION | |
		NONHEME	HEME
Low			
Iron in meat, poultry, or fish	30 g		
Ascorbic acid taken	25 mg	3%	—
Medium			
Iron in meat, poultry, or fish	30–90 g		
Ascorbic acid taken	25–75 mg	5%	23%
High			
Iron in meat, poultry, or fish	>90 g		
Ascorbic acid taken	>75 mg	8%	23%

Treating Anemia   The current standard therapy for iron deficiency anemia is ferrous sulphate administered orally three times daily as tablets, each containing approximately 60 mg of iron. However, Paul R. McCurdy and Raymond J. Dern of Georgetown University (Washington, D.C.) and Loyola University's Stritch School of Medicine (Chicago) have shown how vitamin C aids in iron absorption. They conclude: "The potentiation increases with increasing doses of ascorbic acid. The use of iron preparations containing ascorbic acid may permit the use of less frequent doses in the therapy of iron-deficiency anemia and may refill iron stores better than oral iron salts without ascorbic acid."

OVERLOAD?

All the data point to one conclusion: the greater the vitamin C consumption, the greater the iron absorption. This is "good medicine"—up to a point. Then one needs to ask: Can we take too much C and therefore overload ourselves with iron?
We know of no studies that show if and when such an iron

overload can occur. There are, of course, studies of patients with iron-overload disorders. Siderosis is one. The disease occurs in iron miners and arc welders who, after prolonged inhalation of iron-containing dust, may develop a chronic inflammation of the lungs. Another such disease is thalassemia, a serious and chronic type of hemolytic anemia we described under "Hereditary Disorders" in Chapter 4. Another rare syndrome involves iron-laden pigmentation of the skin, cirrhosis of the liver, diabetes mellitus, and deposits of iron-containing pigments in functional parts of organs such as the liver and pancreas.

Vitamin C to the Rescue

Although no one knows for sure if ascorbic acid could contribute to an iron overload, we know that it can facilitate elimination (as well as absorption). One of the common denominators in iron-overload disorders is the need to get rid of the excess iron. Chelation techniques, intended to bind to the metals and eliminate them, are hampered by limited efficiency of the substances available and by a tendency for them to lose effectiveness with continued administration. The chemical changes required can be facilitated by adding a reducing agent such as vitamin C to the iron chelator being given.

Vitamin C deficiency is common in individuals with iron-overload disorders. A. A. Wapnick from the University of Witwatersrand in Johannesburg (South Africa) decided to find out whether replenishing tissue ascorbic-acid levels would cause increased urinary excretion of iron following the administration of the iron chelator—desferrioxamine. His subjects included twelve with siderosis, thirteen with refractory anemias requiring multiple blood transfusions, eight with thalassemia major, one with sickle-cell thalassemia, and some others with miscellaneous blood-related problems. He also included twelve normal subjects as controls.

Three fairly well established theories were confirmed: vitamin C concentrations in white blood cells are subnormal in people with iron-overload disease; the low C levels are a direct consequence of the excess stores of iron; oral or parenteral (by injection) administration of C results in urinary excretion of large amounts of oxalic acid—an oxidation product of ascorbic acid, which probably undergoes accelerated metabolism because of the massive storage deposits of ferric iron.

When white-cell C was restored to normal limits, desferrioxamine-induced urinary iron excretion increased by 88 percent in thirteen individuals with transfusional siderosis; 60 percent in five with idiopathic hemochromatosis; and a big 350 percent in subjects suffering from the rather rare disease called *dietary siderosis*—which sometimes occurs in people who ingest unusually high levels of iron. At the same time, average white-cell C concentrations rose by 164 percent, 157 percent, and 551 percent in these respective patient groups, which illustrates the tremendous extent of the initial depletion.

Working exclusively with young thalassemia major patients, Richard T. O'Brien of the Department of Pediatrics at Yale University School of Medicine noticed similar improvements. The average desferrioxamine-induced urinary iron output doubled—although there were individual variations, with increases varying between 25 and 200 percent.

C'S DOUBLE ACTION

As the studies we've cited indicate, vitamin C helps people who have too little iron absorb it better and it helps those with too much iron get rid of it.

So how much C should people take for the vitamin's iron connection? It depends on what your iron levels are. This is not a matter for amateurs to pursue. We think it best that people find themselves a competent, nutrition-oriented practitioner who can perform appropriate tests and direct a sensible vitamin C program.

Whatever the extreme—too little iron or too much iron—it seems obvious that the amount of ascorbic acid required is far greater than the so-called RDA. Studies described in this chapter suggest that a daily supplement of from 200 to 1000 mg of vitamin C would vastly enhance iron absorption.

12
A "C" Full of Smiles

Maybe the "glamour" has to to with the gravity of some diseases. Certainly both in TV-land and the real world, little drama is associated with bleeding gums or crooked teeth. Yet more people have a mouthful of health problems than will ever be stricken by cancer or heart disease. And, unfortunately, they can't be brushed away—not even with the fanciest, tastiest, most high-budget-advertised gel or paste.

When the National Center for Health Statistics issued its HANES I report—an acronym for Health and Nutrition Examination Survey—it became part of the record that one out of four adult Americans is minus half to all of his or her teeth! And in older adults who *have* teeth, about 64 percent are afflicted with periodontal disease—inflammation of the gums, periodontal pockets (those nasty cuffs of tissue around the necks of teeth that are associated with the loss of bone support), and a lack of firmness in bony sockets.

These alarming figures are based on an extensive survey conducted in sixty-five locations throughout the United States. And they are most likely on the modest side, since, in order to avoid clinical disagreement, only the most obvious problems were noted under the standardized guidelines used.

Might you belong to the "gum-trouble club?"

Do your gums bleed spontaneously . . . or with eating something like a soft sandwich . . . or a hard apple . . . or during toothbrushing?	YES	NO
Are your teeth loose?	YES	NO
Are your gums occasionally or constantly sore or tender?	YES	NO
Is there bone loss around your teeth as demonstrated by x-ray?	YES	NO
Are there significant pockets around the necks of your teeth?	YES	NO

As we keep emphasizing in this book, *all* disease can be viewed as an interplay among diverse environmental challenges, internal coping mechanisms, and therapeutic aids. It's traditional dental philosophy that the majority of oral problems results from irritants—especially plaque and calculus (tartar). It follows that the solution is to eradicate these troublemakers. But how? Just as one individual may swallow loads of pneumococci "bugs" and never get pneumonia, while another individual gets the disease practically every winter, two seemingly similar people may have the very same amount of plaque. Yet they'll show different clinical pictures of disease in their gums, teeth, the bone surrounding the teeth, and other mouth tissues. The answer must lie in people's differing coping mechanisms, as well as other factors inside the body. For example, Walter Cohen, Dean of the University of Pennsylvania's School of Dental Medicine, showed that adult diabetics suffer more gingival (gum) inflammation than nondiabetics even when they do not show more plaque.

The myth of "great checkups" (meaning no cavities) is slow to die. But it's gory gums that cause the most damage. When pockets deepen, gums recede, and underlying bone gets resorbed (dissolved), one is faced with gum surgery and other periodontal procedures that can cost up to several thousand dollars. Also, teeth may shift around and assume misaligned positions.

Left uncorrected, periodontal disease progresses like a sneaky destroyer. The sequence goes something like this: bacterial colonies grow; pockets are formed in that soft tissue below the gum line; a breakdown in periodontal membrane (fibrous connective tissue around teeth) occurs. As the pockets deepen, the gums recede further; inflammation increases; and underlying bone is resorbed. At this point, the jawbone around tooth sockets shrinks and teeth wobble. Then extensive periodontal treatments—usually involving surgery to remove the pockets and reattach the gums—are necessary to save one's shaky teeth.

TESTING C CONNECTIONS

There are several methods used to analyze vitamin C's connection to periodontal disease. In many experiments, vitamin C is pitted against a placebo, and various measurements of periodontal status—gingival inflammation, tooth mobility, depth of the sulcus (the tissue cuff that surrounds a tooth)—are compared.

In other tests, one side of an individual's mouth receives prophylaxis (cleaning and polishing) and the other does not. Then one-half of the subjects receive C supplements. So we have four possibilities: one side without prophylaxis and without vitamin C; one side with prophylaxis but without C; one side with C and without prophylaxis; and one side with both prophylaxis and vitamin C supplementation.

In a third approach, less widely utilized, the question centers about whether the tartar and plaque might be caused or otherwise influenced by vitamin C.

EXPERIMENTS AND RESULTS

Gummed-Up Gums

Almost two hundred years after Navy Surgeon James Lind studied the vitamin C connection (although he did not call it that), two of his descendant colleagues, F. Stanley Roff and A. J. Glazebrook, worked with a group of sixteen-year-old Royal Navy trainees. For twenty-two days, each subject received 200 mg of vitamin C each day. For the next twenty-three days, they were given

50 mg daily. The incidence of gingivitis (inflammation of the gums) declined 13 percent in contrast with a bare 3 percent in controls. Roff and Glazebrook use a phrase we have used, contending that the marked C deficiency noted by lab tests actually amounted to "subclinical scurvy." And as for there being no way to brush away the offenders, they say: "Marginal gingivitis is due to accumulation of food debris and tartar deposit associated with lack of oral hygiene, and that improvement in personal cleanliness and routine dental treatment will, in the majority of cases, lead to a cure. The most energetic efforts of this type, however, failed to cause any change in the commonest lesion observed amongst these boys, which is a gingivostomatitis *clearly associated with hypovitaminosis C.* For investigations upon actual cases have in every instance shown a deficiency in this factor, and *saturation with ascorbic acid has never failed to effect a cure*" [italics added]. That, we believe, is saying a mouthful for the vitamin C connection to oral-tissue problems.

But that's not the only pro-C mouthful. Emma D. Kyhos and her team at the Department of Medicine at the University of Wisconsin and the Wisconsin General Hospital in Madison wrote: "The most striking observation of [our] entire study was the relationship between the plasma ascorbic acid level and the health of the gums."

In a seventeen-month study of seventy-one male prisoners, Kyhos and co-workers saw gingival improvement increased in direct proportion to the amounts of C given: 25, 50, then 75 to 100 mg.

In an experiment involving 150 male and female personnel in the Royal Canadian Air Force, Major W. J. Linghorne and his colleagues chose participants who exhibited mild to moderate gingivitis. Each subject first underwent local treatment (cleaning and polishing of the teeth) along with instructions for home-care oral hygiene. Then each subject was started on one of four ascorbic-acid dietary regimens:

10 mg per day
25 mg per day (simulating the then-standard civilian average)
10 mg per day plus a 70-mg tablet of vitamin C
75 mg per day

Following another prophylactic session, gum status was graded in terms of gingival bleeding, tenderness, redness, and swelling. Eight months later, the examination was repeated. Readers of this book will, at this point, hardly be surprised to learn that—generally speaking—the greater the amount of C, the greater the degree of improvement.

At Window Nook, Arizona, 168 Navajo students were paired according to age, sex, and gingival status. One group received 300 mg of C daily in tablet form; the other, a placebo. Barbara S. McDonald, a Nutrition and Dietetics Officer of the Division of Indian Health, United States Public Health Service, reports marked gum improvement in the C-supplemented group.

Similar results were obtained in fifty-three dental students observed over a twelve-month period by A. E. Thomas and colleagues at the University of Alabama School of Dentistry in Birmingham. Half the students refrained from taking citrus fruit; the other half received daily supplementation of frozen orange juice. The report says that there was a noticeable worsening of gingival hue (gum color is a good clue to gum health) in the nonsupplemented group and "a significant improvement in gingival hue" in those subjects who drank orange juice.

Another University of Alabama team headed by Gamal El-Ashiry randomly chose subjects who would receive a 100-mg lactose placebo with each meal for twenty-one days, and an equal number who were given 100 mg of synthetic vitamin C at the same mealtime points. Each subject received a thorough scaling of the teeth on one side of the mouth. This matches our "four-possibilities" design described earlier: prophylaxis (cleaning and polishing) with C; no prophylaxis with C; prophylaxis with placebo; no prophylaxis with placebo. Gingival assessment for the twelve front teeth was made before scaling and after twenty days of the C or placebo. Neither the examiner nor the patient was aware of the initial scores or the nature of the supplement.

As one might expect, there was no significant change in the group with no prophylaxis and no C. At the opposite end of the pole, improvement was greatest with prophylaxis plus C—a 58 percent reduction in gingival inflammation. The other two groups also showed improvement, so El-Ashiry and his colleagues conclude that both prophylaxis and vitamin C are valuable tools in combating gummed-up gums, but that the combination of the two works best of all.

The same investigators tested vitamin C versus placebo, with and without oral prophylaxis, on sulcus depth. (The sulcus is the cuff of tissue surrounding each tooth.) With vitamin C alone, the improvement in sulcus depth was 30 percent. With C plus prophylaxis, it was 33 percent.

Sulcular oozing of fluid, along with gingival bleeding, the general condition of gums, and the amount of plaque on the teeth, were measures of oral health or sickness used by R. N. Vest, Jr., and H. Zion in a study performed at the University of Alabama School of Dentistry in Birmingham. The investigation is of particular interest because (1) the experiment was done in a conventional dental setting where vitamin C is not recognized as a factor in gum disease, and (2) it involved the use of the highest amount of C—3000 mg per day—yet reported for oral research.

Subjects were twenty-nine young women and eleven young men all between the ages of twenty and thirty and presumably in good health. Each subject first received a thorough scaling of the teeth on one side of the mouth. Then half the subjects were given 1000 mg of vitamin C three times daily; the remainder, an indistinguishable placebo.

No change occurred in the control group, but the "combined effect of the prophylaxis and vitamin C appeared to be the greatest while the prophylaxis alone and the vitamin C therapy alone yielded essentially the same result."

Periodontal Perils

The periodontal membrane is a ligament between the tooth and the surrounding bony socket. Adrian Cowan (Faculty of Dentistry, Royal College of Surgeons in Dublin, Ireland) studied a group of seventy-eight young patients (average age, twenty-nine) drawn at random from his private practice. He examined approximately 650 tooth roots before and after vitamin C supplementation and compared them versus no supplementation. Cowan states that "areas of irregularity in the [periodontal] membrane have shown an improvement of outline in a significant number of [vitamin C] treated cases as compared with controls in a double-blind investigation." Optimal improvement, as judged by x-ray, was obtained with a vitamin C dose of about 1 gram (1000 mg) per day.

Plaque and calculus add to socket instability and can wreak havoc in terms of periodontal disease. With 108 light calculus formers, 73 moderate ones, and 19 heavy ones, Gilbert Stanton showed that a 500-mg daily dose of vitamin C can keep the calculus away. Each subject was given 750 mg of C for a month and then 500 mg each day for seventeen months. After one year, calculus redeposition was considerably less with many individuals in the light and moderate groups. After about eighteen months, 82 percent of *all* the patients were no longer forming calculus. At the end of the eighteen-month test period, C supplementation was reduced to 100 mg daily. At this level, approximately 75 percent of previous calculus formers remained clear of these deposits. (In a control group, untreated calculus formers remained calculus formers and twenty-three out of twenty-five noncalculus formers showed no change.)

Clearly, swallowing vitamin C can influence irritants inside the mouth. But a group at the Department of Periodontology at the Dental Faculty in Oslo, Norway, decided to study the *local* effect of a vitamin C tablet on plaque formation. Measurements included the gingival index (GI), the plaque index (PI), and thorough prophylaxis to eliminate all calculus and plaque from all the teeth. The subjects (male and female dental students with an average age of twenty-three) were then instructed to discontinue all personal oral hygiene measures for fifteen days. Each participant was next given a coded supply of tablets, to be chewed for one minute four times daily. Results? The vitamin C tablet "showed a statistically significant inhibition of plaque after three and eight days of no oral hygiene."

The same Norwegian research team, headed by Johansen, also checked the effects of this vitamin C tablet—called Ascoal T— when it was used in addition to regular oral hygiene measures. Fifty members of the Royal Norwegian Air Force (average age, twenty-two) participated. Here, too, "Ascoal T had a statistically significant effect on the amount of plaque on the teeth."

"The Barrier Coefficient"   Healthy sulcus epithelial tissue acts as a barrier against microbes and microbial toxins that might otherwise penetrate inward. As gum health worsens, "the barrier coefficient" is lowered—thus the "penetration factor" increases.

In his doctoral dissertation at Massachusetts Institute of Technology, H. M. Mallek showed that vitamin C strengthens crevicular (sulcus) tissue, causing a significant decline in penetrability. He administered 1 gram (1000 mg) daily for four weeks to accomplish these results in eleven presumably healthy seventeen- to twenty-three-year-old subjects.

Tottering Teeth

Tooth mobility is another result of gummed-up gums. The same University of Alabama School of Dentistry group cited previously (headed by El-Ashiry) also studied the effect of ascorbic acid on tooth mobility. Clinical mobility of twelve front teeth was measured on three scales: slight front and back mobility; marked front and back looseness, plus side mobility; marked front and back, along with side and vertical mobility. A mean (average) score was derived from each side of the mouth. Following prophylaxis and C, tooth mobility decreased by 67 percent. C alone—that is, without prophylaxis—netted a reduction of 33 percent. *No* change occurred with placebo, with or without prophylaxis.

Another tooth-mobility experiment was reported by T. J. O'Leary and co-workers. Subjects with wide variations in periodontal health were randomly assigned to four experimental groups: placebo for twelve weeks; placebo for six weeks, then vitamin C for the next six weeks; vitamin C for six weeks, then placebo for six weeks; vitamin C for the entire twelve weeks. The C was administered in a 300-mg capsule each day with breakfast.

Tooth mobility for six upper teeth was measured by a device that records in inches down to the fifth decimal, and these measurements were taken frequently during the course of the experiment. While no statistically significant difference was observed, the researchers explained that the lack of effectiveness of C in decreasing tooth mobility could have been modified by a good preexperimental vitamin C level of the subjects, which had not been taken.

The Crooked Smile

Orthodontics means, literally, "straight teeth." *Malocclusion* means, literally, "bad closing." If you don't have children of your own, ask some close friends what kind of bite orthodontic work takes out of *their* family budget each month. Scoring twelve- to seventeen-year-old youths on the ten-point Treatment Priority Index (TPI, a malocclusion-severity scale), approximately 11 percent of the youngsters in America demonstrate normal occlusion. Some 35 percent show only minor problems. Approximately 25 percent have definite malocclusion, but of a nature that allows straightening procedures to be considered "elective." However, a full 29 percent show very severe handicaps that really demand treatment. In one recent year, it was estimated that 20 million dental visits were made to have teeth straightened. And all these figures apply only to children and adolescents; they do not include the increasing numbers of adults undergoing orthodontic care, not knowing that Tully and Cryer maintain that "the supporting tissues of the teeth may not be healthy," so that results may be compromised.

Where does vitamin C fit? In most orthodontic texts, it is never mentioned. But in the second edition of *Current Orthodontic Concepts and Techniques: Volume I,* Touro M. Graber and Brainerd T. Swain take pains to spell out the importance of collagen and how a deficit of vitamin C may affect it. They state: "This should lead to the conclusion that a high intake of vitamin C is to be recommended for orthodontic patients."

While this conclusion has, so far, found its way into few textbooks, it has—fortunately for people with crooked smiles—been supported by research studies, some of which we'll outline in this chapter.

We set about to test children who were going to have orthodontic treatment. Our subjects were 139 children and adolescents aged 9.2 to 17.6 years. We took the plasma ascorbic-acid level approximately two hours before breakfast and then used ICNND criteria (Interdepartmental Committee on Nutrition for National Defense) to assess vitamin C status. Interestingly, 17.3 percent of this "healthy" group displayed suboptimal C levels, and if one were to use the higher figure of 0.6 mg percent that some authorities feel is more reasonable, 53.5 percent would be considered deficient. Thus, somewhere between one-fifth and one-half of these "healthy" youngsters suffer from a vitamin C deficit that could influence their orthodontic therapy.

Judged by the lingual vitamin C test—remember the experiments measuring how long a blue dye takes to vanish?—these same orthodontic patients displayed even worse vitamin C levels. Some 72 percent (about three out of every four) showed a deficit.

In the previous section of this chapter, we wrote about tooth mobility. Orthodontic movement of teeth causes a significant degree of tooth mobility— a problem orthodontist Emanuel Wasserman investigated in a graduate dissertation. His study involved fifty-one orthodontic patients (thirty-three males and eighteen females) between 12.3 and 16.3 years. In an experimental subgroup of twenty-three patients, eleven maintained their usual dietary intake of vitamin C and took a 500-mg supplement of C each day. The other twelve were instructed to eliminate all foods high in vitamin C, and no supplement was given.

Throughout tooth straightening, there was a significantly greater increase in tooth mobility in the C-depleted patients, nor did mobility return to "physiologic range" after a six-week stabilization period. The opposite was true in the C-supplemented group; still, even they never attained "complete" recovery to the original baseline levels. Our clinical hunch? The 500-mg supplementation was simply not enough.

Root resorption is another orthodontic-related problem. The end of the tooth dissolves and the root becomes thinner and shorter. As long ago as 1940, C. E. Randolph stated that after two years of orthodontic treatment, 75 percent of a patient's teeth show root resorption. As Nathan S. Tom points out, this has made orthodontists wary about injuring roots. They tend to regard root resorption "as a scar from orthodontic treatment, and perhaps as a necessary evil."

Evil, yes. Necessary?

Dr. Tom decided to find out. Orthodontic patients were randomly chosen from those with vitamin C levels rated as marginal to poor (later, additional subjects with satisfactory scores participated in a second study). Other than instructing the experimental subjects to take one 500-mg, time-released vitamin C capsule daily, no special measures were taken.

X-rays were taken at the beginning and at the end of the study. Crown and root lengths were measured, and a proportion technique allowed measurement of the percentage of apical root resorption occurring during the eight-month period. The C-supplemented patients won the contest by a wide margin.

CA/DA/BA

"Stick out your tongue!" used to be—sometimes still is—one of the physician's first commands. Actually, the oral cavity is an excellent barometer of general health or sickness. Also, the eruption schedule of the teeth is one of the most sensitive measures of overall growth and maturity.

Some years ago two of us published two papers dealing with the relationship of chronological age (CA), eruption of the teeth or dental age (DA), and bone age (BA). Subjects were 141 children being readied for orthodontic treatment. DA was determined from x-rays of the teeth. BA was judged by the development of the wrist bones (a standard method). Finally, vitamin C levels were determined by the plasma ascorbic-acid test and by the lingual vitamin C test.

In 88 of the 141 children (62.4 percent), dental age was less than chronological age. It was nearly equal in very few, and higher in only 48 subjects. So we see that—at least in this study— almost two out of three orthodontic patients show delayed dental eruption.

Was this related to suboptimal C? The answer seems to be "yes." We examined lingual vitamin C test times. As lingual times increase, meaning the vitamin C state becomes worse, the correlation between chronological and dental age diminishes. Those children with the most optimal vitamin C levels seem the most "on time" when it comes to tooth eruption. This is very important because the closer these ages are together, the greater the deterrent to malocclusion.

We also found a significant relationship between nutritional status and bone age, and among children's vitamin C levels and CA/DA/BA.

DOES EVERYONE AGREE?

Con

Not all investigators agree—but their studies seem to contain certain peculiarities of experimental design we feel are worth mentioning. For example, W. P. Stamm and co-workers from the Royal Air Force Institute of Pathology and Tropical Medicine studied gingival bleeding in C-supplemented and nonsupplemented personnel. They reported that subjects showing clinical improvement, or no change, or worsening, were similar in both groups. But no data were provided about any measure of tissue-vitamin C state at the beginning. Could the subjects have already had good C levels?

Austin H. Kutscher of the Division of Research, School of Dental and Oral Surgery of the Faculty of Medicine, Columbia University in New York City, reports no difference in clinical response of gingivitis patients receiving 3 grams of C each day versus a control group, even though he does say that "three of the nine improved cases in the vitamin C group showed sufficiently marked improvement as to indicate probable response to vitamin C." Nevertheless, no statistical analysis was included and no blood or tissue C levels were recorded. Perhaps most interesting, the initial "rating" was done during curettage (scraping under the gum line) of one-half the mouth (the upper and lower quadrants on opposite sides). The final rating was done upon curettage of the other, previously unscaled quadrants. So the starting and the final score do not represent the same tissue areas.

At the College of Medicine and Vermont Agricultural Experiment Station, University of Vermont in Burlington, Harold G. Pierce and co-workers used gingival changes as a measure of

ascorbic-acid deficiency. In their student-nurse subjects, they noted some pitting, abnormal color, recession, and blunting and
swelling, but they reported no significant effect of C supplementation on these signs. However, both experimental and control
subjects were said to be in an optimal vitamin C state when the
experiment began. So one would not expect the gingival signs in
these students to respond to C if satisfactory ascorbic-acid levels
already existed.

Finally, Gilbert J. Parfitt and Cletis D. Hand, of the University
of Alabama, worked with twenty male and twenty female institutionalized mental patients. The twenty controls received no vitamin C supplement; the other twenty were given 200 mg after
breakfast, 100 mg after lunch, and 200 mg after dinner. No significant differences in gingival scores were noted. But it should
be kept in mind that a one-month dietary analysis showed a fairly
good vitamin C intake to begin with (167 mg each day). The
other interesting factor is that, even after a daily supplement to-
taling 500 mg, the plasma C level did not rise much. This is con-
sistent with a fact outlined in more detail in Chapter 14: persons
who are psychologically disturbed may require more C because
they tend to excrete too much of the vitamin and its metabolites.

Pro

Fortunately for clinicians, patients, and the public at large, research continues. It's no monkey business that pro-C findings
were reported by Olav Alvares and his colleagues at the University of Washington. They tied silk thread around a single molar
tooth at the gumline of monkeys. In two weeks, compared with
monkeys fed adequate vitamin C, animals with only marginal
intake showed 36 percent greater gingivitis and 41 percent greater gingival sulcus depth.

The study suggests that, as vitamin C dropped, microbe-de-
stroying blood cells could no longer carry out their search-and-
destroy mission *and/or* the deficit in C contributed to gum permeability so that toxic substances could more readily penetrate
the periodontal barrier and cause damage.

Fibroblasts are cells necessary to the manufacture of healthy collagen—that supportive substance mentioned so often in this book. From Temple University's School of Dentistry, Joseph J. Aleo reports that coating fibroblasts with ascorbic acid protects them from endotoxin, which is produced by plaque and microorganisms in the gingival sulcus. These laboratory findings suggest that, when body ascorbic-acid levels are high enough to prevent a deficiency in the gums, these tissues are better able to resist the destructive effect of endotoxin.

KEEPING A BITE IN LIFE

In this chapter we have pretty much ignored dental caries for the simple reason that, compared with periodontal disease and gum problems, it seems rather insignificant. We have also reserved some other oral problems—like wound healing and stomatitis—for other chapters. Still, we feel we've said a mouthful about the connection between vitamin C and keeping a bite in life.

But before we conclude this chapter, let's outline in straightforward, everyday language just a few things that research has shown us vitamin C can do for one's mouth:

It can strengthen the periodontal membrane.
It can reduce gum inflammation.
It can diminish plaque formation.
It can minimize gum swelling and bleeding as well as after-meal brushing can.
It can boost the effectiveness of orthodontic work.
It can *prevent* a need for orthodontics.
It's of cosmetic value because it contributes to pink, healthy-looking gums and straight teeth—in addition to preventing teeth from moving around.

Although a few studies we've mentioned fail to give C an "A," *not one* of them even hints at any harmful effect. Therefore, we see no reason not to recommend vitamin C to any potential member of the "gum-trouble club"—particularly since so much of the research points to remarkably good results.

13
Seeing with C

For a very long time, vitamin A has enjoyed really good press as "the eye vitamin." Some of this publicity is certainly merited, because if vitamin A is lacking, rhodopsin (visual purple)—a light-sensitive substance in the eye's retina—is adversely affected. When this happens, night blindness results.

Night blindness is certainly a serious-enough disorder and one that can prove extremely inconvenient. But it is *blindness itself*—that universally dreaded lowering of the curtain to sight and all it means in our lives—which is of paramount interest and concern when people think of their eyes.

There are, of course, many causes of blindness—systemic diseases like diabetes, certain infections, serious eye injuries, genetic mishaps, and the cataracts associated with old age. However, by far the leading cause of blindness is glaucoma. Here's another area where the vitamin C connection comes in, as we'll see by the research described in this chapter.

EXACTLY WHAT IS GLAUCOMA?

The healthy eye has an optimal or favorable pressure inside it—that is, an *intraocular pressure* that keeps the eyeball from collapsing. Although there is some variation from individual to individual, and even within the same individual from time to time, this pressure remains fairly constant as a result of continual renewal of fluids inside the eye.

Before better education, public-service advertising, TV dramas, and free pressure-measuring examinations made "glaucoma" a household word, the disorder was commonly called "hardening of the eyeball." While there are many types of glaucoma, increased intraocular pressure is the common denominator. And, unfortunately, this "hardening of the eyeball" usually creeps up insidiously—sometimes not being noticed until the visual field has been significantly reduced. On the other hand, there may be warning signals. Check this list to see if you have any.

Do you sometimes see rainbow-colored rings or halos around lights?	YES	NO
Have you noticed a narrowing of your usual visual field?	YES	NO
Have you had frequent changes in corrective lens prescriptions without noticing much improvement in vision?	YES	NO
Do you feel your vision is abnormally poor in dim light?	YES	NO
Have you experienced fuzzy or blurred vision that may come and go?	YES	NO
Do your eyes "water" or discharge fluid?	YES	NO
Do you suffer from vague headaches or eye aches—particularly after watching movies or TV in darkened rooms?	YES	NO
Have you noticed any change in eye color or clouding of the cornea?	YES	NO
When you carefully touch a closed eyelid, do you feel any abnormal "hardness" of the eyeball?	YES	NO
Have any of your relatives had glaucoma?	YES	NO

If two or more of these danger signals apply to you, we suggest that you consult an eye doctor who, in addition to other examinations, will perform tonometry (a painless technique that measures intraocular pressure).

How Can It Be Contained?

Fortunately there are now medicines and also surgical techniques that *control* glaucoma. We emphasize "control" because the medical profession does not regard these measures as a "cure." And in

some people the treatments do not prevent the disease from pro-
gressing. So it is also fortunate that, here too, we have a vitamin C
connection.

Vitamin C to the Rescue   In a Ph.D. dissertation at New York
University, Ben C. Lane established a significant relationship between intraocular pressure and the vitamin C content of diets.
Working with more than sixty subjects ranging in age from twenty-six to seventy-four, Lane found an average intraocular pressure
of 22.33 mm Hg (millimeters of mercury) when daily C intake
averaged 74.6 mg. When daily C intake averaged 1205 mg, intraocular pressure was only 15.15 mm Hg on the average. The
$P < 0.001$ level of statistical significance means that there is less
than one chance in a thousand that the difference could be an
accident—that is, not a result of the vitamin C.

A series of controlled studies was conducted by Professor Erik
Linner of the Department of Ophthalmology, University of
Umeå, Sweden. Both oral administration and topical application
of ascorbic acid resulted in a 2-mm Hg reduction in intraocular
pressure after two days. When the vitamin C was withdrawn, the
pressure rose again.

In one Linner group, twenty-five subjects with moderate ocular
hypertension (another phrase for elevated intraocular pressures)
showed an average pressure drop of 1.10 mg Hg on a regimen of
0.5 grams (500 mg) four times a day for six days. In another
group, a 10 percent aqueous solution of ascorbic acid was applied
three times daily to one eye only for three days. Opposed to the
"control" eye, the vitamin C–treated eye showed an average decrease of 1.19 mm Hg in intraocular pressure. Results of both
were statistically significant.

Extremely encouraging findings were also presented by a team
from the Rome Eye Clinic in Italy, headed by Michele Virno.
They used C doses of 0.5 grams per kilogram (2.2 pounds) of
body weight. Thus, a person weighing 150 pounds would receive
35 grams (35,000 mg) of vitamin C—approximately 600 times the
so-called RDA! The average pressure decrease—16 mm Hg in
two hours—after a single megadose of C highlights the dramatic

findings of this experiment, as summarized in the table that follows.

TYPE OF GLAUCOMA	NO. OF EYES	AVERAGE MAXIMUM INTRAOCULAR PRESSURE REDUCTION (IN MM HG)
Chronic simple glaucoma		
initial pressure 50–69	7	25.0
initial pressure 32–49	7	19.0
initial pressure 20–31	11	6.5
Acute glaucoma		
partial angle closure	3	28.5
complete angle closure	4	10.5
Hemorrhagic glaucoma	2	17.0
Secondary glaucoma	5	11.5

In the normal eye, the average pressure reduction after oral C was 3.5 mm Hg. In general, intraocular pressures reached their lowest point about four to five hours after subjects took a single dose of vitamin C; this low point was maintained for more than eight hours. As one might have predicted, the highest level of blood vitamin C matched the lowest measurements of intraocular pressure.

To counteract the stomach discomfort and diarrhea experienced by some subjects, Virno and co-workers later divided the C dosage into smaller units taken throughout the day.

At the Provincial People's Hospital in Harbin, China, Drs. Tsun-mou Shen and Ming-Ching Yü have been using an intravenously administered solution with sodium ascorbate since 1970, when they found it caused a 20.6–84.2 percent pressure reduction in glaucomatous eyes and a 30.1–64.9 percent drop in the same patients' normal eyes. They noted that the decrease started within fifteen to twenty minutes and progressed to its lowest levels within thirty to sixty minutes.

Here in the United States, Frederick Stocker from the McPherson Hospital and the Glaucoma Clinic of Duke University School of Medicine reports favorably on the pressure-lowering effects of a C-related substance administered to patients with primary glaucoma.

WHAT DOES THE RESEARCH TELL US?

Although Fishbein and Goodstein (Queens Hospital Center, Jamaica, New York) failed to find any positive effect of vitamin C in enhancing the treatment of open-angle glaucoma, most of the work points to a clear vitamin C connection.

Commenting not only on the Virno *et al.* report but also on other investigations done at the Eye Clinic of the University of Rome, Professor G. B. Bietti draws some conclusions that are well worth quoting in their entirety.

1. In large doses, ascorbic acid is a very effective agent for reducing intraocular pressure when administered intravenously (sodium ascorbate 0.4 to 1 gram per kilogram of body weight) or orally (single dose of 0.5 gram per kilogram of body weight or in fractional doses during the day).
2. The pressure-lowering effect of ascorbic acid by mouth lasts longer than that of other osmotic agents given orally or intravenously (including sodium ascorbate).
3. Orally administered ascorbic acid has a varying intensity of action which depends on the individual patients and the type of glaucoma. It is more effective in chronic open-angle glaucoma.
4. It has been demonstrated that the hypotonic action of ascorbic acid on the eye can be prolonged indefinitely, at least for the seven-month period observed here, by administration of 125 milligrams per kilogram of body weight three to five times a day.
5. Normal intraocular tension was achieved with ascorbic acid alone or in association with topical medication (miotics). On some occasions, this happened when miotics by themselves were unable to control the tension.
6. Orally administered ascorbic acid lowers intraocular pressure through several possible mechanisms—an increase in blood osmolarity, diminished production of aqueous by the ciliary

epithelium, the possibility of an improved aqueous-fluid out-
flow or a shift of blood pH toward the acid side.

In short, through one or more of the mechanisms outlined by
Professor Bietti, vitamin C lowers intraocular pressure; it is effective for long periods of time; and it may boost the value of local
medication that's being given for glaucoma.

We feel these facts speak eloquently in favor of C's connection
to seeing.

14

It's *Not* All in Your Mind!

Most people are familiar with the story about two psychiatrists who pass each other in the corridor of a hospital. One says, "Good morning." The other nods but then, continuing to walk, silently asks himself: "What did he mean by that?"

Once a person is steeped in an ethos, it may be hard to react out of character!

Madness has always possessed a certain cachet, frequently being associated with societal preoccupations of the times. It's been variously tied to divine intervention, demons, defective genes, chemical imbalances, evil spirits, the tolls of high technology, and many other factors.

In recent times, the pendulum has swung so widely that a lot of people seem to believe "it's all in your mind." Fanned by the ever-glowing fires of media hype, the news is out that if you're in a bad mood or can't concentrate or are having other mental *or physical* symptoms, it's in your head. The implicit (sometimes explicit) message is that you ought to be seeing a psychologist or psychiatrist—although many people have tried to take matters into their own hands by joining the burgeoning special groups that promise new ways to cope.

Government surveys show that one out of ten adult Americans has had some disorder likened to a "nervous breakdown." More than 17 percent of adult Americans are said to be depressed. Some 14 million people over twenty years of age take sleeping pills from time to time; 6 percent of the United States' adult population take them at least once a week. Possibly most alarming: at any given time, from one-third to almost one-half of all hospital beds are occupied by patients with mental or emotional disorders.

The question is: *Is* it all in your mind?

Ken would not say so. And we believe many people who are equally aware of how much is "out there"—that is, not inside your head—will agree. We've decided to outline Ken's story because so many case histories seem to concentrate on middle-aged, middle-class women, almost as if, disquieting as some of these women's lives may be, men are somehow immune to stressors and their effects.

Ken's rise in the world of high finance had come in steady, step-by-step progression. Friends had to assume that on the job Ken moved with decisive authority. But they frequently noted how at home he was relaxed, informal, easygoing, and devoted to his children—taking time to help them build shadowboxes or whatever the toy of the moment might be.

After years of transferring about the country, Ken and Dora and their children (by now in high school and college) settled down in a fieldstone house in the suburbs of a major Eastern city—satisfied (in their own judgment, that of their kids and friends, Ken's firm, and an interviewing psychologist) that life was good.

Then things started to happen. Within two years, Ken's world fell apart.

Dora contracted a rare form of meningitis. It eluded diagnosis for a while and within weeks Dora was dead.

His only grandchild, the infant son of the daughter who had married a college classmate, drowned in a tragic boating accident that nearly cost the lives of the baby's parents, too.

The middle child, a boy, narrowly escaped death when his motorbike was sideswiped by a large truck. Although he survived, he continues elaborate (and expensive) medical treatment and has not been able to start college.

Ken's father, with whom he shared a warm companionship, collapsed dead, leaving his mother what she herself calls "a nervous wreck."

Substantial damage was done to Ken's house by a freak flood that completely ruined his den and the family room. No sooner had they cleaned out the wreckage than a second flash flood occurred.

But, although his world fell apart, Ken did not. He cried at the funerals; spoke openly of his grief; spent lots of time reassessing his own life and life in general; and methodically set about reordering his financial affairs to absorb Bubby's medical expenses and repair his own water-soaked house. In psychological parlance, Ken reacted "appropriately." One could easily argue that this—as well as other factors, such as an adequate support system (family and friends) and a work life he viewed as satisfying—kept Ken from falling apart.

But there's another factor that is well worth mentioning. From childhood on, Ken had drunk orange juice with every breakfast and often munched on fresh fruit and vegetables. Then, ever since college days—when a football-playing friend started touting the virtues of vitamin C—Ken had faithfully taken *at least* 1000 mg of C every day, and more when he felt under stress or that a cold was coming on.

Could fresh citrus fruit and regular vitamin C supplementation have kept Ken from going bonkers when his world fell apart? No one can be absolutely sure how much each factor might have contributed but, as this chapter will explain, there's a lot of research that supports vitamin C's connection to a person's mental state. Also, there is absolutely no reason *not* to take C, whereas—as we'll see later on—there are 131 lines of small type that tell people why they may not want to take a frequently prescribed "good-mood" pill. We think the evidence speaks eloquently for this C connection and we'd be most reluctant to scoff at the idea that Ken's capacity to cope was tied to his use of C.

But, before we go further, let's check out twelve medical-history questions that are effective in revealing early signs of emotional disturbance. Be honest. Which answers will *you* circle?

Do you have thoughts you can't get out of your head?	YES	NO
Have you felt you were going to have a nervous break-down?	YES	NO
Are you bothered by nervousness and tension?	YES	NO
Have there ever been times when you couldn't take care of things because you just couldn't cope?	YES	NO
Do you have trouble getting to sleep or staying asleep?	YES	NO
Do your hands ever tremble enough to bother you?	YES	NO
Are you ever disturbed by nightmares?	YES	NO
Are you troubled by your hands' sweating?	YES	NO
Have you ever fainted or blacked out in recent years?	YES	NO
In the past few years, have you had frequent headaches?	YES	NO
Have you ever had spells of dizziness?	YES	NO
Are you bothered by your heart beating hard?	YES	NO

A U.S. Public Health Service report shows that 78 percent of the adults examined in a National Health Survey answered YES to one or more of these questions. The average was 2.29. But "average" need not be "healthy." If you have circled a couple of YESes, you may find this chapter of special interest.

PSYCHE AND SOMA

Some Outmoded Ideas

For a while there it looked as if psychosomatic medicine might sweep the field: mind over matter. The notion was that "life upstairs" (the *psyche*) had such an all-powerful influence over our body (the *soma*), that it could generate all sorts of bodily ills. To some, this seemed to mean *all* bodily ills. At the same time, the mind could "cure" all sorts of diseases, or control pain.

It's clear that the mind can exert quite an influence. In Chapter 16, we'll see how—in part—a positive attitude helped writer-editor Norman Cousins through his illness. And Dr. Norman Vincent

Peale's books contain literally hundreds of stories about the "power of positive thinking."

The problem? It seems that much less attention has been paid to the *soma-psyche* side of mental well-being, that is, how physiological disruptions might fire off "bad signals" to the brain and cause perceptual or conceptual distortions that can cause abnormal behavior.

There was an era, too, when *projection* was held to be the key to jarred thinking and erratic behavior. The whole "projective technique" in diagnosis was based on the premise that, given an ambiguous stimulus (like the Rorschach Ink Blot Test or the TAT, standing for "Thematic Apperception Test"), an individual will "project" his or her own way of seeing the world. However, up until around the early 1960s, few researchers had set about to show that there might be a certain stimulus pull in the tests themselves. If this is so, it is not all in the subject's mind; some of what emerges is right there in the test instrument—which calls into question many aspects of projective theory. We did some work in this area, not only with a rarely used projective test (which would seem to suggest that the more commonly used ones are open to even greater question) but also with patients for whom the process of group therapy was materially influenced by *commonly shared* interpretations of drawings they made. Another experiment on perception showed how external events mold imagery of stereotypes.

In short, mental-health professionals are now less sure that they are working on a one-way street, psyche to soma, or soma to psyche; inside one's head to outside in the world, or outside in the world into one's head. Once again, *active interplay* between and among various forces seems to hold the key. Let's see how vitamin C may play an important role in all this.

Some Facts About C

The brain is not just a skull-encased control center that is somehow separate from the rest of the body. Nor is the nervous system merely a complex set of switches and tracks that relay messages back and forth—brain to body, body to brain.

The brain and the nervous system are an integral part of one's total body. As such, they must constantly be nourished by oxygen, by glucose, and by many other nutrients, including vitamin C.

But the nutritional needs of brain and other nerve cells are unique. To illustrate this point, suppose you could capture the amount of energy consumed by the human brain in twenty-four hours. This "fuel" would suffice to heat half-a-dozen quarts of water from freezing to boiling!

Mother Nature seems to have recognized nerve cells' special need for vitamin C, for the level of ascorbic acid is considerably higher in cerebrospinal fluid than in blood plasma. In subjects with plasma C levels of 0.68 mg percent or more, the cerebrospinal fluid:blood ratio was 3.28:1. Even in those with levels less than 0.68 mg percent, it was 2.04:1. Vitamin C's concentration in the brain exceeds that in any other organ except the adrenal glands. The adrenals, as biology students know, are tied in with reactions of the sympathetic division of the autonomic nervous system, which stimulates reactions to emergency stress.

Research with lower animals suggests that C's entry into the central nervous system is regulated by a kind of transport system in the choroid plexus—a series of folded, membranous structures where the fluid-filled chambers of the brain meet those of the spinal cord. These controlling mechanisms allow brain cells to be bathed with C-rich cerebrospinal fluid. This continues even when dietary intake or blood ascorbic-acid levels drop. However, only a small quantity of any oral dose of C crosses into the brain, so supplementation is desirable to ensure preventive and/or therapeutic levels of this essential brain metabolite.

MOOD, MIND, AND MENTAL HEALTH

Recent Research

In this book we frequently describe how vitamin C improves people's sense of well-being. It seems to work against anxiety, tension, pain, and other stresses. Now let's see how some studies over the past couple of decades have shown vitamin C's connection to mental health—even though we realize no one has yet precisely defined just what "mental health" (or "mental illness") is!

Report Summaries   Humphrey Osmond (a research psychiatrist at the University of Alabama in Tuscaloosa) and Abram Hoffer (a psychiatrist in private practice in Victoria, British Columbia) describe ascorbic acid as a natural internal tranquilizer. That is, it counteracts anxiety. In fact, these researchers contend that, weight for weight, ascorbic acid "is as active as Haldol." This is quite a statement, for Haldol is a major tranquilizer— "major" differentiating it from the "minor" tranquilizers that are often (possibly too often?) prescribed to help people cope with the stresses of everyday modern life. However, lest a reader worry about overmedicating with C, remember that, as Drs. Osmond and Hoffer emphasize, only a very small amount gets to the brain, and *no one* has ever found that vitamin C worsens any condition.

There's no doubt that vitamin C can also help people withdraw from tranquilizers. In the next chapter, we'll outline this action in more detail. For the moment, let's just mention the Stoke Park Hospital (Bristol, England) study conducted by J. Jancar. More than half the C-supplemented patients remained off tranquilizers, with no unpleasant effects, over a two-year period. Perhaps this is because, as Osmond and Hoffer observed in schizophrenics and G. J. Naylor saw with manic-depressives, ascorbic acid itself offers relief from anxiety and tension. Indeed, Osmond and Hoffer's patients responded to daily 10-gram ascorbic-acid doses when no tranquilizer had been helpful. Naylor's subjects (under the tight controls of a double-blind, placebo-matched, crossover trial) showed significant improvement in only two days after a *single* 3-gram dose of C.

How Might C Work?

There are three ways of looking at relationships between a person's vitamin C status and his or her psychologic health. In scientific assessment, each of these approaches is valuable. We'll describe some research that flowed from each viewpoint.

The Symptom-Free Subject   We used the Cornell Word Form-2 (CWF-2) to screen out "mentally healthy" subjects who scored either 0 (136 people) or 1 (148 individuals). These subjects—as well as more than 200 who scored higher figures (in more "pathological" ranges)—were then analyzed by food-frequency analysis and a seven-day diet diary. Computerized results provided a rundown of the daily intake of all major food categories—protein, carbohydrate, and fat—as well as vitamin and mineral intake.

The seven-day dietary survey showed that subjects with CWF-2 scores of 0 took in 148 mg of C daily; those scoring 1 (or more) consumed 128 mg. These average values were statistically significant at the $P < 0.005$ level. The food-frequency questionnaire showed an average daily C intake of 294.9 and 249.9 mg, respectively. (These figures are higher because this technique also allowed inclusion of supplementary C that was taken.) Here, too, there was a highly significant difference: $P < 0.005$.

What this means is simple: the higher the C intake, the lower the incidence of psychological problems—*even* in the two groups considered to be "well glued together" in comparison to those with higher CWF-2 scores.

The C-Deficient Subject   Another method involves assessing behavioral and emotional symptoms in subjects with and without a vitamin C deficiency.

Myron Brin described five stages in the progressive depletion of a nutrient. Without intervention, severe clinical deficiency and death result. Brin says that "marginal vitamin deficiency states correspond to the first three stages of deficiency and *behavioral changes are likely to be among the consequences of marginal vitamin deficiency*" [italics added].

In an experiment at the U.S. Army Medical Nutrition Laboratories, volunteer subjects took the Minnesota Multiphasic Personality Inventory (MMPI). Those suffering from marginal deficiency of vitamin C showed MMPI profiles with significantly increased hypochondriasis (an unfounded belief one is suffering from disease), depression, and hysteria.

Progressive Development of Vitamin Deficiency

DEFICIENCY STATE	SYMPTOMS
1. Preliminary	Depletion of tissue stores (due to diet, malabsorption, abnormal metabolism, etc.). Urinary excretion depressed.
2. Biochemical	Enzyme activity reduced due to co-enzyme insufficiency. Urinary excretion negligible.
3. Physiological and behavioral	Loss of appetite with reduced body weight, insomnia or somnolence, irritableness, adverse changes in Minnesota Multiphasic Personality Inventory scores.
4. Clinical	Worsened nonspecific symptoms plus appearance of specific deficiency syndrome.
5. Anatomical	Clear specific syndromes with tissue pathology. Death ensues unless treated.

Controlled Therapeutic Trials As we've explained before, correlation does not necessarily mean cause-and-effect. One would need to test C versus a placebo in emotionally disturbed patients. Milner's study at Towers Hospital in Leicester, England, did just that. In a controlled, double-blind study, Dr. Milner worked with forty male chronic psychiatric patients. Half were given 1 gram (1000 mg) of ascorbic acid each day; half were given a placebo.

While Milner used the term "subscurvy" rather than "marginal deficiency," his subjects could be classified as being in the first three stages of Brin's scheme.

With C saturation, over a six-day period, statistically significant improvement was noticed in the instance of depressive, manic, and paranoid symptom complexes, together with an overall improvement in personality functioning. Both the MMPI and the Wittenborn Psychiatric Rating Scale were used in the evaluations.

Dr. Milner says: "States of depression and anxiety associated with psychiatric disorders are probably accentuated by an inadequate intake of ascorbic acid." He also suggested that "chronic psychiatric patients would benefit from the administration of ascorbic acid."

This latter recommendation is strongly supported by the findings of T. P. Eddy, reported in more detail in Chapter 2 of this book. Dr. Eddy investigated the woeful state of food served in hospitals: in psychiatric hospitals the average daily vitamin C totals only 21 mg. That might suffice for an adult guinea pig but it comes nowhere near what's needed by an adult human being!

Mental Performance

The old nature-versus-nurture controversy has threaded its way in and out of prominence in the psychological literature ever since the field first emerged as separate from philosophy, cultural and biologic anthropology, sociology, and other disciplines in its heritage. Sometimes in vogue and sometimes out of vogue, the controversy keeps reemerging because—in all truth—no one has satisfactorily answered questions about the relative importance of each.

However, one major aspect of the environment has received little consideration when it comes to the nature-nurture dispute: *diet and nutrition.* Albert L. Kubala and Martin M. Katz at the Department of Psychology at Texas Woman's University decided to see if citrus-products deficiency might have any effect on mental-test performance.

Subjects from three schools ranged in age from preschool classes through the ninth grade. On the basis of blood-plasma ascorbic-acid levels, each subject was assigned to a "high" (1.1 mg percent or more) or a "low" (less than 1.1 mg percent) group. Subjects within a given school system, but divided into one of the two C-intake groups, were matched by a series of socioeconomic indicators and IQs. The latter were determined by examinations with one of the Pintner tests or the Otis Quick-Scoring Mental Ability Test, according to the subject's age.

In all schools, mean or average IQs fell as follows:

High C	113.22 IQ
Low C	108.71 IQ

The difference was statistically significant at $P < 0.05$, which means in less than 5 cases out of 100 could this be accidental.

The researchers then sought to see if daily C supplementation in both of these groups with a large glass of orange juice would have any effect. The initially high-C group remained about the same, but the low-C group benefited: there was an increase of approximately five points in average IQ.

Children from the two elementary schools were tested a total of four times during the experiment. On each occasion, the change in mean plasma ascorbic-acid level and the change in IQ closely paralleled each other.

The findings are especially interesting when one realizes that Kubala and Katz called less than 1.1 mg percent "low" but not "deficient." Currently, plasma C levels as low as 0.2 mg percent still escape the "deficient" label as set by government standards. To quote no one in particular: "How low do you have to sink?"

A PILL VERSUS A PILL

Although we find research reported here—as well as other investigations—quite encouraging, we are *not* claiming that vitamin C will put a definitive end to all emotional or mental difficulties. Nor do we say it will put psychiatrists and psychologists out of business; turn your child from "normal" to "bright normal"; or totally revolutionize therapeutic approaches.

What we *are* saying is that C has some definite connections with mood, mind, and mental health; that both clinically and experimentally it has been shown to be of benefit; and, in contrast with some pharmacologic agents, *it does no harm.*

If we were showing slides, the point would emerge in almost awesome graphics. Since this is a book, we must ask our readers to use a little imagination and make a comparison between a frequently prescribed "minor tranquilizer" (Pill 1) and a tablet of vitamin C (Pill 2).

If you consult a recent edition of *Physicians' Desk Reference,* the guide most widely used by practicing physicians and those in training, you will find the following information about Pill 1 (the minor tranquilizer).

CATEGORY	LINES OF SMALL TYPE
Contraindications	8
Warnings	24
Psychological and physiological dependence	22
Usage in pregnancy (warnings)	17
Management of overdose	17
Precautions	22
Adverse reactions	21
Total	131

And what have we under Indications? That is, for what symptoms might one prescribe the drug? Here we have twenty-six lines of small type. In short, there are five times as many reasons *not* to prescribe the drug as there are reasons a doctor might wish to prescribe it!

Contrast this with vitamin C (Pill 2). In not one reference guide we know of is there even a single contraindication, warning, precaution, or note about dependence, overdose, adverse reaction, or any problem in pregnancy. And the indications? Count them from this very book. Since we have zero (0) against, we can't come up with a multiplication factor! Let's just say the score is 100 percent pro against 0 percent con.

15

Addiction Plus Vitamin C
Equals No Addiction

In the last chapter, we mentioned that just as vitamin C can act as a tranquilizer, it can also help people to withdraw from such drugs.

The public may prefer to view great scientific discoveries as coming from dedicated, white-coated researchers bent over their laboratory tables. But often scientists, however dedicated and however white-coated, may mimic "The Three Princes of Serendip" by accidentally finding the unexpected by happy accident. Two well-known examples of serendipity occurred in the laboratories of Wilhelm Konrad von Roentgen and Dr. Alexander Fleming.

When Professor Roentgen passed electric charges through a high-vacuum tube covered by black cardboard, he noticed a green glow coming from a small object on a neighboring bench. He then tried other opaque objects, such as a big fat book, and also his own hands. Some unknown ray—thus, the name x-ray—penetrated each item and left an "interior" image on paper that had been coated with a certain chemical.

Thirty-four years later, in 1929, a mold floating about the damp air of Paddington Station drifted through an open window of Fleming's laboratory and lighted on an exposed culture plate. The mold devoured colonies of staphylococci and, after further observations, Sir Alexander predicted that someday *penicillin* "would come into its own as a therapeutic agent."

Slightly more than forty years after that time, Ewan Cameron and G. M. Baird set about to see if they could duplicate other experiments that had shown vitamin C useful in treating cancer.

What they actually found was that it (also) works against opiate dependence.

Their subjects were more than one hundred cancer patients, many of whom were ravaged by metastases (spreading) to various body sites. Five of these individuals had been on large doses of opiate painkillers, such as morphine or diamorphine, for some time. "One patient with multiple spinal and thoracic cage metastasis, was inadequately controlled on a dose regime of 30 mg. morphine sulphate intravenously every 3 to 4 hours."

Cameron and Baird reported that within only five days to a week of ascorbic-acid treatment, four of these patients were painfree and the fifth "required only mild analgesics for comfort . . . [and] not one . . . experienced any withdrawal symptoms or made any requests that his opiate regimen should be continued."

The researchers believe that "large doses of ascorbic acid should relieve the physical cause of pain from expanding bone metastasis by retarding tumor growth"—a subject we covered in Chapter 6 and especially in Chapter 10. But what about the withdrawal connection? Being "unable to offer any explanation for the dramatic and unexpected relief from opiate dependence," Cameron and Baird comment as follows: "We believe that this clinical observation from the field of advanced cancer merits further investigation, and *may prove to have practical application in the treatment of opiate addiction*" (emphasis added).

Fortunately, we have reports of "further investigation." Before we describe these research findings, let's pause to define addiction.

ADDICTION: DRAWING THE LINE

Most authorities will agree that addiction can be defined as the *compulsive* use of chemical agents that are clearly harmful to the person, to society, or both. These chemical products have as a common denominator the ability to influence the nervous system in a generally pleasurable manner. An individual quickly learns to appreciate these pleasurable effects so that, after a while, it becomes difficult if not impossible to quit using the drug. Dependence assumes the characteristics of a basic drive, such as hunger or sex. In fact, clinical and experimental evidence makes it clear that addiction actually supersedes both hunger and sex, which makes for further nutritional problems in the addict and further relational problems with the addict's mate.

The drug abuser rarely realizes when he or she becomes an addict. The craving is irresistible, and anyone who has attempted to overcome a relatively mild form of drug dependency—like smoking—knows about those dark and impelling forces that slumber beneath the conscious level of our volitional selves.

In the public at large, addiction is often viewed as a symptom of maladjustment—some psychological disturbance or possibly the acting-out of a social grievance. As Nils Bejerot (Research Fellow in Drug Dependence at the Department of Social Medicine in the Karolinska Institute in Stockholm) explains, drug *abuse* often is a symptom of maladjustment. But, when *addiction* sets in, that in and of itself becomes a pathological condition—with its own special characteristics and its own dynamics.

For example, most adult cigarette smokers are not suffering from a personality disturbance or profound underlying social problems. (As one of our colleagues likes to put it: "Smokers may be 'crazy' but they're not *crazy*.") They probably started smoking as teenagers, imitating elders and wanting to look and act grownup badly enough to hack through many packs before getting hooked. The original reason for smoking (being grownup) has long since passed. But nicotine dependence turned a symptom (wanting to look big) into a disease (poisoning one's own body). That's the way of addiction: it is bound to develop if certain substances are administered in certain quantities over a certain period of time.

RECENT RESEARCH

C to the Rescue

It was actually before Cameron and Baird's report that J. Jancar of the Stoke Park Hospital in Bristol, England, worked over a two-year period with fifty-seven severely retarded males ranging in age from twenty to sixty-three years. These individuals had been taking various tranquilizers for an average of six and a half years.

Leaving other prescribed drugs unchanged, Dr. Jancar planned a tranquilizer-withdrawal program over a three-month period, replacing tablet for tablet with 50 mg of ascorbic acid. This phase was followed by three months of gradual withdrawal of the C, then an eighteen-month observation period.

At the end of the entire trial period, thirty (52.6 percent) of the fifty-seven patients remained off tranquilizers, with no side effects. Of the twenty-seven patients who had to be placed back on tranquilizers, twenty had physical or mental disorders superimposed on mental retardation. Only nine of the thirty people in the "success" group had such ailments. We would speculate that, with larger doses of vitamin C, more if not all of the fifty-seven patients could have been freed from tranquilizing medications.

Not long after the Cameron and Baird report, Jordan Scher and a group of investigators from the National Council on Drug Abuse and the Methadone Maintenance Institute in Chicago told a gathering of the North American Congress on Alcohol and Drug Problems that vitamin C can reverse side effects in methadone-maintained patients. (Methadone has been widely used to wean addicts from heroin, but the drug creates its own addictive problems.) The researchers showed that daily administration of 5000 mg of vitamin C relieved three complaints: constipation, reduced libido ("sexiness"), and restless sleep. During the three-year treatment period, other annoying side effects of methadone treatment were eliminated: "Many methadone patients will show low-grade irritability, discomforting emotionality, debility and mood shifts. After vitamin C, these patients will seem to feel an enhanced sense of comfort and well-being."

In Scher's double-blind (neither party knows) study of addicts undergoing drug withdrawal and detoxification, those who received a daily 5-gram (5000 mg) dose of vitamin C rather than a placebo showed marked relief from fatigue, tension, disturbed sleep, muscular pains or cramps, vasoconstriction and cold limbs, constipation, and impotence.

Some Theories   Scher and co-workers are convinced vitamin C is effective; they say it "is an excellent addition to the armamentarium of narcotic-addiction treatment on a clinical and statistical basis." While they are not certain of the pharmacologic and biochemical principles behind C's action, they believe that it works as a physiologic tranquilizer and might be employed to replace other, stronger and less physiologic tranquilizers.

Alfred F. Libby and Irwin Stone have another theory. They believe that some people are born with a genetic defect when it comes to metabolizing vitamin C. The problem continues throughout childhood and on into later life. The "faulty genes" theory could explain why already-low body stores of C are depleted even further as the addict loses his appetite for food.

Libby and Stone also contend that providing a high dosage of vitamin C can immediately detoxify a drug so that no high occurs even if the addict sneaks a fix during treatment.

Two Detox Programs   For Libby and Stone, treatment consists of giving patients from 25 to 85 grams (note, that's grams, not milligrams!) of sodium ascorbate each day in spaced doses, along with high intakes of other vitamins, essential minerals, and predigested protein. This schedule is continued for four to six days. Then doses are gradually lowered to a holding level of from about 10 to 30 grams each day. (Specific amounts vary from individual to individual, with bowel tolerance as one criterion.) During the megadose phase, no withdrawal symptoms should be encountered. If any appear, the sodium ascorbate is increased.

Improved mental alertness and visual acuity, along with increased appetite and feelings of well-being, are noted within only twelve to twenty-four hours after the sodium-ascorbate detoxification program is begun.

Translating high doses of vitamin C into "street terms," a $50 habit requires approximately 25 to 40 grams (at a C cost of $1.25 to $2); a $150 to $200 habit requires about 60 to 75 grams (a C cost of $3 to $3.75).

Similarly encouraging news comes from the San Francisco Drug Treatment Program. In a search for safer and less-costly detoxification alternatives, several unconventional approaches were tried. Valentine Free and Pat Sanders investigated using vitamin C megadoses in conjunction with multivitamins, minerals, and protein supplementation in treating drug-withdrawal symptoms.

All 227 participants received a routine physical examination, as well as a checklist that covered the daily recording of symptoms the individual noted (subjective) and those an interviewer observed (objective). The list included common signs such as runny eyes and nose, sweating, chills, muscular aches and pains, diarrhea, abdominal cramps, drug craving, loss of appetite, sleeping difficulties. Each client met regularly with an assigned counselor who dealt with clinical issues, and all subjects followed a twenty-one-day detoxification plan.

The big difference was in the C.

Group I received 24 to 48 grams of sodium ascorbate or ascorbic acid every twenty-four hours for five to seven days, tapering to 8 to 12 grams for fourteen days. (Multivitamin and multimineral tablets, calcium complex and magnesium, and liquid protein were also given.)

Group II received symptomatic relief medications—propoxyphene hydrochloride, Belephen, Librium, and, at bedtime, chloral hydrate.

Group III received a combination of the two regimens.

The results are summarized below.

Average No. of Withdrawal Findings

| | TIME PERIOD | | |
	AFTER 1 DAY	AFTER 1 WEEK	AFTER 3 WEEKS
Group I (C)	6.5	3.0	2.0
Group II (medications)	8.0	8.0	6.5
Group III (C & medications)	9.0	1.0	1.0

In the overall sense, the combination approach showed the greatest reduction in symptoms—although, initially, the vitamin C program seems to be most successful. Certainly both in terms of patient comfort and cost effectiveness, the use of vitamin C warrants much more investigation—particularly because it could be administered in outpatient settings.

REHABILITATING REHABILITATION

In the majority of drug-rehab programs, the addict is subjected to a curious twist of logic: he (or she) is transferred from an "illegal" hard drug such as heroin to a "legal" hard drug such as methadone. Actual withdrawal and reentry into a drug-free existence are goals eluded by many addicts and almost ignored by some rehabilitation personnel. Since vitamin C offers the possibility of a simple, safe, inexpensive, and healthy solution to the problem, we believe more widespread use and study should be welcomed, encouraged, and pursued with vigor.

Nor do we believe that research should be confined to opiates, tranquilizers, and heroin or methadone. We'd like to see serious scientific investigations of how vitamin C might help smokers, overeaters, heavy drinkers, and other addicts kick their habit.

16
Plugging in More Connections

Up to now we have discussed many health problems that a hefty amount of scientific research has shown are connected to deficits in vitamin C. There are others for which the connection is less well established, yet evidence points to some potentially important relationships. We would be remiss not at least to mention some of these investigations, even if more thorough scrutiny is in order.

SOME BEGINNING LOOKS AT C-ING

Much of the work grouped in this present chapter might be characterized as "preliminary reports." Most of the investigations were conducted quite recently and not one of the studies predates the 1960s. We applaud these pioneering efforts to extend vitamin C's many connections and we eagerly await further research in these areas.

A Brief Rundown of Various Studies

While the number of these research studies is somewhat limited, the C connections are positive. Not a single report contains a "negative" note suggesting that ascorbic acid might worsen some disorder. So we are convinced that these findings should be brought to the broader public. Purely for reader convenience, we'll outline research results under names of disorders or subjects listed in alphabetical order.

Ankylosing Spondylitis and Viral Encephalitis   Norman Cousins—Editor Emeritus of *The Saturday Review* and internationally respected as a modern-day version of the Renaissance man—fell ill with a crippling and supposedly fatal disease. The diagnosis: ankylosing spondylitis, a collagen disorder in which connective tissue disintegrates. In the best-selling *Anatomy of an Illness*, Cousins describes his struggle to take responsibility for his own life. He chose to shun traditional medical approaches in favor of massive doses of ascorbic acid—which his scientific reading had indicated served as a regenerative agent in conditions similar to his—along with an attitude of positive reasoning, spirited humor, and the stimulation of books, movies, TV, music, and good friends.

His recovery sparked world-wide interest, ranging from doctors to lay people, to specialists attending a conference in the Soviet Union, to the lawyer-father of a four-year-old girl stricken with viral encephalitis. Rebuffed by physicians who refused to consider the lawyer's collection of pro-C medical papers published in Europe, the young man decided to take matters into his own hands. He mixed at least 10 grams (10,000 mg) per day of ascorbic-acid powder with his daughter's ice cream, and he saw remarkable daily progress.

After the little girl's recovery, Cousins asked the lawyer if he had told the medical specialists what he had done. "Certainly not," he replied. "Why should I make trouble for myself?"

As Norman Cousins put it: "One can understand the apprehensions of the medical profession about the absurd notion that vitamins are the answer to any illness. Yet it is also true that some doctors have fostered the equally erroneous idea that the average supermarket shopping basket is insurance against any nutritional deficiency."

Cousins contends that his "cure" resulted from a combination of many things, including mental attitude and vitamin C. A lot of professionals would probably argue that his positive mental state was the key. Yet was the little four-year-old girl capable of exerting "positive thinking" and enriching her life with good reading, good music, and good friends?

We cannot say for sure what role vitamin C played in these two "miraculous" recoveries, but we find it impossible to believe that it played no role at all, especially when we consider all the positive evidence presented throughout this book. We might add that Cousins holds a philosophy professorship at UCLA's School of Medicine and has been active at Columbia University's College of Physicians and Surgeons.

Arthritis   Well over 30 million Americans—about one in seven persons—suffer arthritis severely enough to seek medical help to the tune of 10 percent of all visits to physicians. More than 7 million individuals are disabled, and each year the disorder saps about 27 million lost working days and a combined medical and lost-days bill of over $13 billion. And this $13 billion does not count all the money spent on various nonprescription remedies.

There is osteoarthritis (which generally comes along about the time we get gray hair), rheumatoid arthritis (a systemic disease that also afflicts sites other than the joints), and gouty arthritis (said to be tied to "high living"—especially the consumption of rich meat, alcohol, and sugar). Each of these disorders (and other types of arthritis) is different, but for our purposes here let's simply describe how a joint normally works. A joint, of course, is a junction where bones meet—or let us say *nearly* meet. For the space in between contains a fibrous capsule that encompasses the joint. Inside this capsule is a delicate, wet, velvetlike lining called the synovium. The synovium produces synovial fluid, a lubricant that keeps bones from "rubbing." Sometimes the synovium is inflamed and the victim suffers swelling, redness, heat, and pain. Sometimes a chemical imbalance causes excess uric-acid deposits in a joint. Sometimes the general wear and tear of living to middle age and beyond takes its toll on joints punished by a variety of motions and injuries. Anthropologic digs have shown that not only human beings but also various animals have suffered from osteoarthritis since prehistoric times—even dinosaurs had osteoarthritis!

In a report presented to an International Congress of Rheumatology held in San Francisco, H. J. Mankin of Massachusetts General Hospital called attention to "the fact that the cartilages' response to degradation is replacements by new tissue." Why does this work in some people and not in others? Almost two hundred years after Naval Surgeon James Lind published his findings, Dr. B. E. Ingelmark showed that the amount of collagen—the principal portion of the white fibers of connective tissue, cartilage, and bone—is directly dependent upon the amount of protein *and vitamin C available*. In Chapter 6 we quoted some comments James C. Greenwood, Jr., made about his experiments with using C to combat bone pain. He also reports "more experience since [that time] with many other patients suffering from osteoarthritic problems." Can C stimulate the body's natural effort to repair degraded tissues, to encourage collagen formation? Dr. Greenwood states: "I have seen remarkable results when certain measures are applied—and with them, large doses of vitamin C because vitamin C is very much involved in virtually all body repair processes."

Long recognized for his contributions to neurosurgical and microsurgical techniques, James Greenwood is the Chief of Neurosurgery at Texas Methodist Hospital and Clinical Professor at Baylor College of Medicine in Dallas. So these encouraging words about vitamin C's use in arthritis are *not* coming from a faddist.

Chlorinated Water   Chlorine may be great in swimming pools or for whitening clothes. It is also effective in killing off waterborne microorganisms—which is why it is so commonly used in municipal water supplies. The problem? Not only does it make some faucet water almost impossibly nasty to drink but it also can cripple red blood cells (RBCs) so they cannot carry adequate oxygen around the body.

The problem was solved by John Eaton and his University of Minnesota associates when they determined why patients at two of the three artificial kidney centers in Minneapolis were developing severe anemia. Water used in the blood-cleansing kidney machines was not chlorine-free. Adding vitamin C to the dialysis water neutralized the chlorine. What does this have to do with chlorinated drinking water? The Minnesota researchers advise: "Put vitamin C in your water before you drink it. . . . It's odorless and tasteless in the tiny amount needed—just a trace—to neutralize the chlorine . . . and vitamin C works very rapidly."

Fertility Why are the ovaries so highly endowed with vitamin C? Possibly the "wisdom of the body" is at work! In any event, Masao Igarashi (Department of Obstetrics and Gynecology, School of Medicine, Gunma University, Maebishi, Japan) kept the C connection in mind when he set about to treat forty-two women with different kinds of ovarian problems. Some were anovulatory (no fertile eggs) and some were amenorrheic (no menstrual periods).

Clomiphene citrate, a popular fertility drug, had failed. When vitamin C was added to the clomiphene regimen, 40 percent of the women began to ovulate and 21 percent later became pregnant. Doctor Igarashi observes that "the possible site of action of ascorbic acid seems to be at the ovarian level."

How about men? Impotence has often been tied to "depression, stress, or other psychological factors." At Beth Israel Hospital in Boston, Richard F. Spark and his colleagues screened levels of the male hormone, testosterone, and discovered that suboptimal ranges were also tied to other hormonal imbalances. Once these imbalances were corrected, potency was restored in 90 percent of the patients.

But hormones do not come from thin air. Could there be a C connection? In our own laboratory we pursued this question. We noted the plasma testosterone levels in thirty-six presumably healthy doctors who were taking less than 200 mg of vitamin C daily and compared them with levels from fifty-two presumably healthy doctors who were taking more than 200 mg of C each day. The higher-level-C subjects showed more than a threefold testosterone level: an average of 407 mcg percent (micrograms percent) versus 116 mcg percent.

Growth Many studies show that Japanese-parented people born in the United States are taller than their counterparts in Japan and—perhaps more interestingly—exceed their parents' height to significant degrees. So there must be more to growth than heredity. Is there a vitamin C connection?

Working with eighteen male and twenty-six female pairs of school-age identical twins—that is, offspring developed from the same egg—Judy Z. Miller and co-workers from the Department of Medical Genetics at Indiana University School of Medicine, the Eli Lilly Company, and the Department of Human Genetics of the Medical College of Virginia set to work. Commenting on the male group, the researchers report that "in all but one pair the treated [500 mg of C daily] twin grew from 0.64 to 2.54 cm more than the untreated co-twin during the five-month study period." This result suggests the possibility that C supplementation can help a child grow as much as an inch in five months.

Indigestion The flood of TV commercials for indigestion remedies points to the prevalence of minor gastrointestinal upsets. Over a three-year period at the Monash University Department of Medicine and Prince Henry's Hospital in Melbourne, Australia, J. Hansky and Fiona Allmand studied ninety-three patients admitted for more serious gastrointestinal conditions involving blood where it shouldn't be—in stools or being spit up. By means of several sophisticated diagnostic tests, these subjects were divided into several categories: thirty-seven with duodenal ulcers: twelve with gastric ulcers; nine with hiatal hernias (a condition in which a body structure bulges through the esophageal opening of the diaphragm); four with gastric carcinoma; and thirty-one in whom the site or source of bleeding could not be established. Detailed dietary histories were taken, and these factors were compared with a sex-and-age-matched group of hospital patients with no GI disorder.

In thirty-four of the ninety-three patients with GI bleeding, daily vitamin C intake was under 50 mg. Only fourteen of the control group had a similarly low intake. In the ninety-three GI-bleeding subjects, a history of heavy use of analgesics (pain relievers, such as aspirin) was obtained in seventeen—only three of whom had a low vitamin C intake.

Here's fertile field for further investigation: ascorbic-acid deficiency may be an important factor in gastrointestinal bleeding, and taking supplements may also offset certain painkillers' erosive effects on the GI tract.

Lifespan Throughout this book we talk about how vitamin C can help in scores of disorders, diseases, and health problems. But the bottom line is: Can a C deficit affect one's lifespan?

We have seen that hospitals have a miserable record of dietary practices, and we know that the elderly in institutions (as well as at home) are often malnourished. But the deficiency is not confined to the old—and it can even be influenced by external situations, such as the season of the year, or by internal choices, such as smoking.

T. S. Wilson (Barncoose Hospital in Redruth, Cornwall, England) decided to see if vitamin C levels can be related to death itself among hospitalized patients. He analyzed white cells and platelets for vitamin C levels and found, after four weeks, that the lower the level, the higher the death rate. Expressed another way, the higher the C level on admission, the greater the patient's life expectancy. Wilson's findings are summarized in the following table.

Mortality at Four Weeks After Admission

AVERAGE WHITE BLOOD CELL AND PLATELET LEVEL OF VITAMIN C (MCG)	SAMPLE SIZE	NO. OF DEATHS	MORTALITY (%)
<12	32	14	47
12–18.5	38	14	37
18.6–25.0	40	10	25
>25.0	49	5	10

Dr. Wilson's population sample was selected at random and was highly representative of total admissions for that period. Survival did not appear to reflect any specific clinical features of any particular illness. Could administration of vitamin C materially influence the outcome—that is, life or death?

More study is needed. However, one seminal research project suggests that vitamin C not only prolongs life but also enhances its quality. Several scientists from the Department of Chemical Pathology at the University of Leeds (England), headed by C. J. Schorah, studied 118 long-stay patients aged fifty-nine to ninety-seven. After blood and plasma C levels were determined, subjects were assigned to experimental (vitamin C solutions supplying 1 gram per day) and control (placebo) groups. Various physical measures (such as weight) were made, along with continuing assessment of what many hospital personnel call "activities of daily living." The researchers reported that "the placebo group tended to deteriorate during the trial . . . there were significantly more clinical improvements and weight gains in the vitamin C groups . . . than in the placebo groups. . . . Our results [despite low levels of statistical significance] suggest the need for further and more detailed studies of the clinical and biochemical effects of vitamin C in small and large doses in elderly people in and out of institutions. Similar studies would be justified in younger long-stay inpatients who also have low concentrations of vitamin C in plasma and leukocytes."

Occupational Hazards   What is a worker to do if he is allergic to materials he must handle? Tom (not his real name) suffered a severe dermatitis of the hand. It came from handling chromium-containing inks. Oral antihistamines and corticosteroids didn't work, and he was not able to use gloves or barrier creams. Above all, Tom could not afford to quit his job.

John E. Milner, from the Division of Occupational Medicine of the Department of Environmental Health at the University of Washington in Seattle, reports that a locally applied 10 percent solution of vitamin C did the trick for Tom. The solution altered the chemical structure of the chromium and provided an inexpensive, easy-to-use, safe treatment method. Tom's speedy recovery permitted continued, long-term employment in the field he knew best.

Dr. Milner's report is not alone. From the Department of Dermatology at the Hospital of the University of Pennsylvania in Philadelphia, M. H. Samitz says that 10 percent aqueous vitamin C offers protection from inhalation of chromic-acid mist when the solution is placed into the filters of respirators. Here, too, the mechanism is the alteration of chromium's chemical structure (from hexavalent, or six-pronged, to trivalent, or three-pronged).

These are important findings because, although chromium is best known for its use in electroplating other metals, it is also present in cement (thus affecting construction workers, artists, masons, and tile setters) and in printing inks (so that there is a kind of world-wide epidemic of dermatitis among lithographers).

Skin Problems Approximately one out of every eight or nine Americans suffers skin problems—some 25,218,000 cases in the civilian, noninstitutionalized population of the United States.

Clearly, skins are not clearing under traditional dermatologic therapies. Recalling some diet-identified discussion of "bad skin" in a 1946 textbook by Urbach and LeWinn (*Skin Diseases, Nutrition and Metabolism*), we used a food-frequency questionnaire and the Cornell Medical Index Health Questionnaire in an effort to sharpen the relationship suggested. Our subjects were 1058 doctors and their spouses. In 799 subjects who reported no skin problems, daily vitamin C intake was 335 mg on the average. In 266 persons with one or more skin complaints, the average C per day was less.

We decided to test, over a one-year period, what effect might follow from altering the amount of C taken. In one group, 281 subjects increased their daily C from 240 to 428 mg, average. The decline in skin problems per subject went from 0.47 to 0.27. That is, a 78 percent rise in C resulted in a 43 percent decline in skin problems. By contrast, for the 85 subjects who did not increase their C, or took less—an average decrease of from 416 to 327 mg per day—skin scores at the beginning and at the end of the period were 0.42 and 0.43. In percentage terms, a 2 percent increase in skin symptoms and signs accompanied a 21 percent decrease in vitamin C.

Tay-Sachs Disease This inherited disorder, named for two turn-of-the-century researchers, is a tragic blow to parents and their stricken children. It involves the nervous system, causing blindness, brain pathology, and mental retardation.

Until recently, it has been considered a hopeless and inevitably

fatal disease. But in the late 1960s research work with hexosaminidase isoenzymes—normally present in the human spleen—suggested a remedial approach. Following the discovery reported by
Robinson and Stirling, Shintaro Okada and John O'Brien demonstrated that the activity of one of these enzymes (hexosaminidase
A, or HEX-A) is lacking in Tay-Sachs disease. These findings,
replicated by other researchers, suggested a means of diagnosing
the disease prior to birth. This would allow high-risk parents to
know if their child was going to be normal, but it left no viable
option to couples who might not be willing to abort an affected
fetus.

Perhaps adequate therapy is on the way. Edward Cotlier and
Arlene Duwelius of the University of Illinois studied the effect of
vitamin C on the formation of HEX-A in "normals" and in patients with Tay-Sachs disease. Their conclusion: "the potential
usefulness of ascorbic acid in generating hexosaminidase-A in
vivo is self evident."

White Blood Cells   In several other sections of this book—
especially in Chapter 3, "How Not to Be Bugged by Infections"—we have outlined how white blood cells cruise about the
body looking for "foreign enemies" to destroy. When white blood
cells get sick, we get sick. When enough of them die, we die. In
fact, some seriously ill people succumb not directly because of
their illness but because so many high-powered medications interfere with the vital functions of the white blood cells.

But is there also such a thing as *too* high a white cell count?
Back in 1975, A. B. Robinson, J. R. Catchpool, and Linus Pauling
suggested that increasing C would reduce the *abnormally high*
white-blood-cell counts that accompany many serious disorders.
We undertook to see what relationship C intake and total white-
cell count might show in a reasonably large sample of presumably
healthy subjects.

In 1043 subjects, we noted the daily C range from a low of 15
mg to a high of 1120 mg; the average was 330 mg. Total white-
blood-cell count spread from a low of 3500 to a high of 16,800;
the average was 6598 per cubic centimeter (cc). As we slowly
increased the daily amount of ascorbic acid, both the high and

the low white-cell counts dropped out. Our final average: approximately 5000 per cc.

In short, vitamin C can help when there are too few white blood cells and when there are too many.

SOME CLOSING LOOKS AT C-ING

Here and in earlier chapters we have outlined clinical and research findings that point to vitamin C's connections with numerous states of health and illness; with mental well-being; and with helping in withdrawal and recovery from abused substances. In the next three chapters readers can find out about their own status—how much C they need, whether they can hurt themselves with too much C, and why they should not live by C alone (regardless of how "miraculous" the vitamin may seem).

At this point we merely want to remind readers once again of the enormous number of ailments that respond positively to vitamin C and the fact that not one study shows that it adversely affects the course of an illness. We believe that the public has a right to have this information, a self-help obligation to learn more, and the freedom to choose nutritionally oriented health professionals who will help them apply the knowledge.

17
How Much C Do I Have?

By this time, the reader will probably want to know just what his or her own vitamin C status is. Unfortunately, short of having yourself locked up in the metabolic ward of a hospital, there seems to be no perfect method. Even the metabolic ward—where intake, excretion, and various body levels of C are meticulously determined—is not readily available except for research purposes.

Fortunately, there are ways to get some inkling of your C state strictly on your own, although the assistance of a dietitian, nutritionist, or nutrition-minded doctor can help when it comes to asking the right questions and making accurate interpretations.

Whatever the method used, assessing a person's C status can easily become a matter of life and death. If you doubt this claim, read what Charles E. Butterworth, Professor and Chairman of the Department of Nutritional Science at the University of Alabama in Birmingham Medical Center, had to say about "marginal deficiencies" at a symposium called "Vitamin Nutrition Issues."

Let me begin by citing an isolated case report which I hope will serve as a frame of reference for the identification of marginal deficiencies in the outpatient population. . . . Mrs. S., age 65, was admitted to the hospital for elective pelvic surgery aimed at eradicating recurrent cancer of the cervix. During surgery there was excessive bleeding into the abdominal cavity and surrounding tissues. She required multiple transfusions. In retrospect, it was learned that she had ill-fitting dentures, lived alone, and ate only soft, well-cooked foods. She had consumed no fresh fruits or juices, no raw or lightly-cooked vegetables, and had received no vitamin supplements for over three months. With this background we drew a blood vitamin C level and found it to be in the scurvy range. She died ten days later of cardiopulmonary arrest. . . . My purpose in giving this account is to suggest that the marginal deficiency in this woman might have been recognized by an interview with a dietician and a laboratory screening program. . . . Unfortunately, very few clinics and hospitals are set up to provide such a service."

From this one might conclude: Well, gang, you're on your own! And, to a large extent, this is true. Below, we have divided discovery techniques into two groups: do-it-yourself and where a professional might be necessary or helpful. But the groupings are rather arbitrary. For example, a dietitian or nutritionist can be of great help when you want to interpret a dietary review. On the other hand, a lay person, good at interpreting tables, might do his or her own dietary history or food-frequency questionnaire. Certainly most people can use C-Stix.

So the reader should keep in mind that there's a lot of "back-crossing" in our division and that, generally speaking, we prefer to recommend consulting with nutrition-minded health professionals when it comes to tests and interpretations.

SOME TECHNIQUES FOR DISCOVERY

Do-It-Yourself

Questionnaires   While the questionnaire review approach is the least sensitive of measuring sticks, it is clearly the simplest and the cheapest. Simply flip back through your own answers to the questions we've posed in most chapters of this book. If you have lots of YES answers, you can be reasonably sure your vitamin C level leaves much to be desired.

Dietary Reviews   In their book *Cancer and Vitamin C*, Ewan Cameron and Linus Pauling list the vitamin C content of 110 raw natural plants and the concentration of C per 2500 calories of food energy. (That's the average daily energy requirement for most adults.)

"Super-high" C foods include broccoli spears, black currants, kale, parsley, hot chili peppers (red and green), and sweet peppers (red and green).

"High" C foods include Brussels sprouts, cabbage, cauliflower, chives, collards, and mustard greens.

"Intermediate" C foods include artichokes, asparagus, beet greens, cantaloupe, chicory greens, Chinese cabbage, fennel, lemons, limes, oranges, radishes, spinach, zucchini, strawberries, Swiss chard, and ripe tomatoes.

Here's a useful list.

FOOD	MG OF C
⅖ cup frozen concentrate orange juice	229
⅖ cup frozen concentrate grapefruit juice	138
1 large green pepper shell	128
1 cup cooked Brussels sprouts	135
1 stalk raw broccoli	113
1 cup fresh orange juice	124
1 cup fresh lemon juice	112
1 cup fresh grapefruit juice	95
1 cup cooked collards	87
1 orange	80
1 cup raw cauliflower	78
1 cup cooked turnip greens	68
½ raw cantaloupe	63
10 whole raw strawberries	59
1 carton raspberries	59
1 avocado	43
½ raw grapefruit	38
¼ honeydew melon	35

Keep in mind, however, as we described in Chapter 2 ("Vitamin C's 'Vanishing Act'"), these figures are based on food-composition tables and are significantly inflated over what's left after the total garden-to-gullet preparation that so often ends in *over*cooking.

Other foods are lower in C, but are often eaten with considerable frequency. So they tend to contribute C by quantity rather than by inherent content. A list of them follows.

FOOD	MG OF C
1 wedge watermelon	30
1 cup lima beans	29
1 cup blackeye peas	28
1 cup dried uncooked peaches	28
1 tangerine	27
4 ounces calves' liver	25
1 cup raw diced pineapple	24
1 raw cucumber	23
1 cup canned pineapple	22
1 baked potato	20
1 head lettuce	18
1 banana	12
1 raw onion	11
4 raw radishes	10
1 cup steamed eggplant	8
3 ounces raw clams	8
1 artichoke	8
1 celery stalk	4
10 potato chips	3

If you're not consuming generous amounts of foods from these two groups or not taking supplements, it is likely your vitamin C state is suboptimal. If you also answered YES to a number of questions in this book, there's even more proof.

Best-Get-Help Approaches

The Dietary History   The dietary history provides what might be termed "presumptive evidence." It cannot spell out your nutritional state with real accuracy, but, if qualifying factors are absent and your nutritional needs are average, it can offer a good gauge.

Once the record has been gathered, the data must be evaluated by a knowledgeable individual. Such an interpretation embraces two phases: determining the nutrient value of the food taken in and interpreting whether it is appropriate for the person.

Precise accounting is difficult to achieve and this, along with differences of opinion about food composition tables, has led to more and more interest in programming computer systems to process such data.

The Food-Frequency Interview   As the name suggests, this technique concentrates on the frequency with which certain foods are eaten: the number of times during a week, or the number of days per week a particular food is eaten. Since common foods are already programmed into the computers, frequency is multiplied by the known composition of the foods. Frequency data have also been correlated with diverse health parameters such as hemoglobin, physique, serum protein, the presence of rheumatic fever, and skin signs of malnutrition.

In our own laboratory, we have experimented with various refinements of this technique and concur with J. H. Abramson and his colleagues at the Hadassah University Hospital and Medical School in Jerusalem. They contend that the method "continues to merit consideration in epidemiological studies" and that it "may be of particular use in the 'clue-seeking' stage."

Biochemical Tests   For definitive assessment of a person's vitamin C state, one must reckon with a variety of processes: absorption, assimilation, utilization, and, finally, excretion of indigestible end products of foods.

For research, these tests can use exotic media such as tears and saliva; for more common purposes, technicians usually measure the C content of urine, whole blood, blood serum and plasma, or tissues such as white blood cells, platelets, and skin.

Because there is a relatively rapid passage of C immediately after intake, urinary excretion is not always the best measure of nutritional state. But, when the tissues are saturated with C, a larger percentage (as high as 60 to 80 percent) can be recovered. So the technique is widely used to evaluate the "load" of C being administered and the number of days required for saturation. Still, interpretation requires caution. For example, one 1000-mg C tablet taken once daily will net greater urinary C than 500 mg taken twice daily. In addition, other non-C factors may affect urinary C excretion.

Commercial tools are readily available. For example, C-Stix consists of a strip of firm plastic material, like a matchstick. It contains a reagent that tests for C in the urine. Once the reagent area is dipped into fresh urine and immediately removed, it can be compared with bottle-label color blocks that reflect 0–10, 25, 50, and 150 mg percent. Without C supplementation, the average range is about 2 to 10 mg percent. With habitual use of large amounts of C, it may rise to 200 mg percent.

This test is most significant when it is negative—that is, showing no C in the urine. This means that the body's need for C has increased and most likely is not being satisfied by the amount that is taken in. The test must be viewed as a crude determinant, which more closely parallels dietary intake than nutritional state.

As the observant reader will have noticed throughout this book, blood is frequently used to measure vitamin C levels. This might involve whole blood, the liquid portion or plasma, or the white cells and platelets. Or serum may be used. When blood is removed from the body and allowed to stand, a clot forms and the liquid that exudes from the clot is called *serum*.

The most accurate blood estimate of C in the body tissues is found by examining white blood cells and platelets in a technique that involves the so-called "buffy coat."

The significant correlation between dietary intake and plasma levels of ascorbic acid has been known for many years. With total C deprivation, the plasma falls to 0 after about 41 days—although it takes about 134 days for scurvy signs and symptoms to appear. However, the zero point is not reached for about 121 days in the "buffy coat" layer. Thus, in terms of namable pathology, the latter material may be the superior indicator. Most authorities believe that the best method lies in examining leukocytes and platelets. Unfortunately, the technique is difficult. Once the blood sample is centrifuged, red cells, which are the heaviest, settle at the bottom of the tube. The plasma rises to the top. Just above the heavy red-cell layer is a thin foamy layer: the "buffy coat," which contains the leukocytes and platelets. It is not easy, even for the most skilled technician, to reach down with a pipette past the plasma layer but not into the red-cell zone to siphon off the leukocytes and platelets.

The Skin Test Plasma levels are an obvious chemical index of how much C is in the circulating blood. Authorities are somewhat less sure about exactly what the skin test—also called the intra-dermal decolorization test—is measuring. But tissue *ought* to provide an even more constant measure since, as we've seen, plasma levels can fluctuate considerably. The intradermal test is calculated to measure ascorbic-acid function at the cellular level, by quantifying the duration and intensity of a deficiency state.

Here's how the test is done. The forearm is cleansed with 70 percent alcohol. A 4-mm area is then marked off with a red pen. With a sterile 2-cc tuberculin syringe and a 25-gauge needle, 0.5 cc of the dye solution is injected between the layers of the skin. This produces a wheal 4 mm in diameter. A stopwatch is immediately set, and the wheal is checked periodically to determine the time required for complete decolorization. The higher the C level, the shorter the time. Less than twenty minutes is considered desirable; twenty to thirty minutes is marginal; thirty to sixty minutes is unacceptable.

While we are among investigators who have used this technique in experiments reported in this book, we admit to its problems: it hurts, it may take an hour, and it is not effective in dark-skinned individuals.

The LAAT, or Tongue C Test   The lingual ascorbic-acid test, also called the tongue C test, is accurate, rapid, painless, inexpensive, and allows for easy correlation and validation. As far as we've been able to determine, fifty-six papers have been published describing experiments in which the LAAT was used, and at least fifty-three of these reports regard the test in a positive light.

How simple is this procedure? The subject is seated in an area where the tongue can be directly illuminated. After the mouth is thoroughly rinsed with tap water, the protruded tongue is grasped with a gauze pad. Another pad is used to dry an area about one-third of the way in from the tip of the tongue. The technician takes care to stroke the hairlike papillae so that they stand erect. One drop of blue dye—2, 6, dichloroindophenol sodium salt solution—is deposited through a 25-gauge needle. The instant the drop lands on the tongue, a stopwatch is started and the time it takes for the blue color to disappear is recorded in seconds. An LAAT time of twenty seconds or less suggests that the tissue is well supplied with vitamin C; twenty to twenty-five seconds is marginal; any value greater than twenty-five seconds indicates a definite deficit. Actually, as a hedge against stress and for quick recovery from trauma or illness, an LAAT time of 15 seconds or less is preferable.

In Krakow, Poland, Giza and Weclawowicz established a clear relationship between LAAT results and the actual liver concentration of vitamin C in women undergoing abdominal surgery. And in our own laboratory we have found statistically significant relationships between LAAT scores and plasma ascorbic-acid levels, nonfasting serum cholesterol levels, and various oral parameters of health and illness. More information about this simple but sophisticated test can be obtained from Medical Diagnostic Services, Inc., Post Office Box 1441, Brandon, Florida 33511.

IS "GOOD" GOOD ENOUGH?

Quite apart from the effects of living habits like smoking and disease states such as impaired intestinal absorption, even adequate dietary intake does not ensure that the body tissues can and will receive a satisfactory amount of ascorbic acid.

Too, food-composition tables can be confusing. Widdowson and McCance of Cambridge University's Department of Medicine put it this way:

> There are two schools of thought about food tables. One tends to regard the figures in them as having the accuracy of atomic weight determinations; the other dismisses them as valueless on the ground that a foodstuff may be so modified by the soil, the season or its rate of growth that no figure can be a reliable guide to its composition. The truth, of course, lies somewhere between these points of view.

The tests we've outlined should take most of the guesswork out of "How Much C Do I Have?" In the next chapter, we'll try to answer the natural follow-up question: "Now that I know how much I have, how much do I *need*?"

18

How Much C Do I Need?

In the last chapter we outlined various methods of assessing your own vitamin C state—or at least taking most of the guesswork out. That *ought* to provide an answer for how much you really need. But does it? Read on!

THE RECOMMENDED DIETARY ALLOWANCE

We've mentioned "the recommended dietary allowance" or RDA many times in this book, often making the point that, for reasons explained and on which we'll expand later in this chapter, we believe it is far too low.

The RDA originated back in 1943 as a "guide for planning and procuring food supplies for national defense." Although the Committee on Dietary Allowances of the Food and Nutrition Board has since then issued new reports at about five-year intervals, we would question the latest official statement that RDAs are selected "on the basis of available scientific knowledge." The latest figures follow.

AGE OR CONDITION	VITAMIN C (MG/DAY)
0–1	35
1–10	45
11–14	50
15+	60
Pregnancy	80
Lactation	100

If one studies the growth rate and other indexes of optimal health in our friend the guinea pig—who, like us, cannot synthesize vitamin C—the creature's ideal daily C intake would be 3.5 *grams* (not milligrams) were he the size of an average man.

But perhaps "optimal health" has little to do with the so-called RDA. the committee itself says: "Special needs for nutrients arising from such problems as premature birth, inherited metabolic disorders, infections, chronic diseases, and the use of medications require special dietary and therapeutic measures. These conditions are not covered by the RDA."

Readers of this book will immediately recognize that this list of "conditions" seems to be much too restrictive. Indeed, it is probable that ordinary, everyday experiences of living in today's fast-paced modern world pose "conditions" that demand a greater need for vitamin C.

But, for the moment, let's return to scurvy—that exotic disease thought to be conquered, but which turns out to be far more prevalent than had been thought. The committee itself says that "a daily intake of 60 mg of vitamin C [that is, the RDA] would be required to maintain an ascorbate body pool of 1500 mg [which] will protect against overt signs of scurvy in the adult for a period of 30–45 days."

What happens after that month or month-and-a-half? Echoing the observations of many other investigators, Robert E. Hodges and co-workers conclude: "The minimal amount of ascorbic acid necessary to prevent or cure scurvy appears to be slightly less than 10 mg daily." But, again to quote the Food and Nutrition Board, that amount "does not provide for acceptable reserves of the vitamin [and] may not be satisfactory for the maintenance of optimal health over long periods of time."

If we need x amount to keep us from getting scurvy, y amount to maintain good general health, and we use up z amount each day by combating stress, indulging in certain living habits, or because we have some "condition" (ranging from low income to a diagnosed ailment), *how much vitamin C do we* really *need?*

"CONDITIONS" THAT WRECK AN RDA

Low Income

Ever since the early 1800s, more and more data have been accumulated and published relating income level to variations in health. Unsurprisingly, chronic disease is more prevalent among low-income populations. On measures of disability, difference by income is quite clear. The number of work-loss days is substantially higher. Yet these figures are most likely *understated,* since many low-income people hold jobs that do not offer sick leave, so these individuals may be forced to work when they're ill rather than lose a day's pay. Fewer medical services are available, and many low-income people rely on hospital emergency rooms and public clinics for such health care as they receive. Further, various sociologic and psychologic factors may add to the burdens of economic want.

A "Vital and Health Statistics" report called *Health Characteristics of Low-Income Persons* calls this population "disadvantaged in health" and estimates their numbers at some 48 million. Clearly, these are people for whom the concept of RDA (let alone higher levels) has little meaning. Also, this report is more than a decade old. How many more individuals have joined these ranks, especially when one considers the vicissitudes of inflation and erratic employment patterns?

Chronic Diseases

Health-survey results are often underreported. Respondents to health interviews may report only conditions they know they have and/or are willing to report. Nonetheless, another U.S. Department of Health, Education, and Welfare publication (also from back in the 1970s) tabulated the prevalence of metabolic disorders and chronic conditions of the genito-urinary tract, nervous and endocrine systems, and blood and blood-forming systems. Some 3 million Americans are suffering from chronic thyroid problems of one sort or another. Diabetes afflicts more than

4 million. Collectively, all anemias total approximately 3 million instances. Migraine headaches afflict about 4.5 million people. Neuralgia, neuritis, and other nonspecific nerve disorders afflict over 1.5 million Americans. All urinary diseases of a chronic nature involve almost 6 million individuals. Disorders characterized as "female difficulties" (but discounting breast disease) afflict some 3 million more. The report sums up: "The 28 chronic conditions groups indicate an estimated 28,245,000 conditions among the civilian, noninstitutionalized population." An additional survey from the same era states: "Nearly one-third . . . or an estimated 60.6 million of the U.S. population . . . have some skin pathology—one or more significant skin conditions that should be evaluated by a physician."

So we have almost 90 million Americans beset with chronic disease—and that does not take into account the *many* disorders that were not included, and the fact that these figures have not been updated!

What this means is that probably one-half our entire population is suffering from "chronic diseases," a category for which even the committee says the RDA is not sufficient.

Medications and "Drugs"

We've already discussed the widespread use of aspirin, and how it has a devastating effect on vitamin C state. The same goes for sleeping pills, contraceptive pills, and the hundreds of prescription and over-the-counter drugs that the public consumes on a regular basis.

Caffeine has a similar action, and back in the 1970s a government survey showed adult consumption of coffee to average 3.2 cups per day among 80 percent of the population. Mothers usually will not allow their children to drink coffee, but they may not think of forbidding carbonated drinks, that contain about the same amount of caffeine as coffee.

Then, of course, we have the smoker. Every cigarette wipes out about 25 mg of C. Hence, all other things being equal, the pack-a-day smoker requires 500 mg more C than the nonsmoker. That amounts roughly to about six tall glasses of fresh orange juice daily or 500 mg of C supplementation.

Thus, if you smoke, drink coffee, and take pills—not even to mention drinking alcohol or taking potent medications—you, too, "are not covered by the RDA."

Eating Patterns

Primitive people even up to the present time "munch" throughout the day rather than confine themselves to fixed mealtimes. Paul Fabry and his research colleagues in Czechoslovakia have confirmed that spaced eating is more effective in providing optimal amounts of vitamin C–rich foods without overloading the system at one time and depriving it at the next. Subjects were divided into several groups and fed precisely the same food, but under different time and quantity schedules. There is absolutely no question but that as one eats less per unit time (smaller meals) but more times per day (except for a heavy bedtime snack, which is harmful) health improves. Dr. Fabry and his co-workers showed that, under such a dietary regimen, high blood glucose levels decline (which invites less diabetes), weight is lost, and serum cholesterol concentrations are reduced.

The harried and hurried, up-and-down eating patterns of many contemporary Americans makes them, too, noncandidates for the RDA.

Individual Differences

Tall people, short people, overweight people, and skinny people all require different-sized clothing. A strapping two-hundred-pound lumberjack needs a caloric intake different from a dainty one-hundred-pound manicurist.

We find it extraordinary that the proponents of the RDA seem not to recognize the importance of individual differences. The celebrated professor and vitamin researcher Roger Williams has shown that, by any number of physical measurements, people can differ by two- to several-hundredfold. Absorption, assimilation, utilization, and elimination of various foodstuffs all differ markedly for different people.

It is simply not possible to come up with a magic daily C intake that will work for every individual adult.

HOW HIGH TO GO?

As we've outlined in this chapter and detailed throughout the book, there are many reasons for believing that the "optimal" daily human need for vitamin C is probably much higher than suggested by the Food and Nutrition Board.

How much higher should it be?

Some investigators recommend a daily intake of around 250 mg. That is about four to five times the present RDA. Others suggest from 5 to 10 grams (5000 to 10,000 mg) daily. That amounts to 80 or as high as 160 times the present governmental suggestion.

We see yet another possibility. It's incontestable that different people consume different amounts of ascorbic acid. One could plot a daily consumption line that goes from zero to tremendous quantities. It's also a well-established observation that some individuals seem to be blessed with no health problems while others appear to be almost allergic to life. Here, one could plot a line of clinical symptomatology ranging from zero on upward.

Could there be a parallel between these two facts? We thought this would make for an interesting and possibly fruitful experiment. So along with Ms. Medford, we examined 1038 presumably healthy doctors and their spouses in terms of ascorbic-acid consumption. Determinations were made by using one of the many—and none is perfect!—food-frequency questionnaires. The one we used evaluates C intake from both foods and supplements. Clinical state was graded by means of the Cornell Medical Index Questionnaire.

The CMI scores, representing the total number of symptoms and signs, were compared with C intake.

There was a very wide range in both measures. Working from the hypothesis that relatively symptomless and sign-free persons are healthier than those who have symptoms and signs, we examined subgroups that could be regarded as being progressively healthier. For example, we reexamined the 1015 persons with fewer than fifty clinical problems. Then we restudied the C intake in the 986 individuals with fewer than forty signs or symptoms. And we went on—under thirty, then under twenty. Obviously, since no one is absolutely "perfectly healthy," one sooner or later runs out of people. But, before that happened, a clear trend crystallized. As we progressively constructed a healthier group, the average daily C intake increased to approach around 500 mg.

From these data, one could say that the so-called RDA should be roughly 8 times what it is. Yet, because the perfectly healthy person living under perfectly ideal conditions is probably a figment of the imagination, we calculate that the *ideal recommended dietary allowance* (which we've come to call IRDA) should be from 1 to 3 grams per day—that is, 1000 to 3000 mg.

If you feel cheated because we are not giving you an exact figure, remember that you are an individual—extraordinary, unique, not quite like any other person. You wear your own shoes, your own clothes, and have your own attributes and foibles. You also know how circumstances can change for you. Thus, you may know when to alter your C dosage just as well as you would know not to wear a cross-country skiing outfit for a summer swim.

You have two options.

First, you can prescribe for yourself—arriving at your decision on the basis of published evidence. Second (and we think the better alternative), you can customize the treatment by consulting with a nutrition-oriented health professional.

19
Can Vitamin C Hurt You?

There's a sentence that appears fairly regularly in the *Physicians' Desk Reference* when that guide describes so many of today's drugs: "The precise mechanism of action has not been clearly established."

Also, if you will turn back to Chapter 14, under the section called "A Pill Versus a Pill," you'll find a rundown on how one popularly prescribed drug—a minor tranquilizer—rates 131 lines of small type devoted to contraindications, warnings, precautions, adverse reactions, and other reasons a doctor may wish not to prescribe it and a patient may wish not to take it.

Yet few professionals or lay people seem to take issue with how "established" drugs work, or what the potential severity of their side effects may be. Nor do they seem to question the alacrity with which federal agencies often approve the marketing of drugs that have not been subjected to maximal testing.

What's the connection? To make headlines, positive data on some beneficial effect of vitamin C would have to be replicated by at least a dozen scientists using long-term, double-blind, crossover studies on thousands of subjects. But newspapers across the nation prominently featured the findings of an undergraduate research project at the University of the Pacific's Department of Biochemistry. The claim was that vitamin C tablets may decompose into products capable of causing diabetes, kidney stones, lactose intolerance, and overweight. The rebuttal by Hoffmann-La Roche (a major producer of vitamin C) did not merit such attention. This happened even though "Stability of Vitamin C Tablets, Fact or Fiction" cited evidence by DeRitter and co-workers, H. S.

Rubin, and many others attesting to C's stability, and even though the report points out that the California researchers only *assumed* oxalate was present in aging vitamin C tablets (they never actually measured it!).

Many researchers (such as A. B. Hanck, Korner and Weber, Cedric Wilson) and many clinicians (such as Frederick Klenner and other doctors cited throughout this book) have administered large doses of vitamin C to large groups of people over extended periods of time. They all concur that, as Korner and Weber put it, there is "no indication of any effect prejudicial to health caused by vitamin C even if administered in high doses."

Nonetheless, some investigations have suggested that large daily doses of ascorbic acid can be dangerous. Since recent surveys indicate that about two-thirds of Americans use vitamin and mineral supplements, we believe it is only fair to outline some of the studies that call vitamin C's safety into question.

Here, too, we are presenting the subjects in alphabetical order purely as a matter of convenience.

B_{12} AND G-6-PD DEFICIENCIES

Vitamin C users are becoming somewhat more used to, and more skeptical of, anti-C news. But back in 1974 they were shocked when Victor Herbert and Elizabeth Jacob (Columbia University's College of Physicians and Surgeons and the Bronx Veterans Administration Hospital) reported that 500 mg of C or more daily can cause a B_{12} deficiency anemia. Lowered B_{12} levels were said to cause shortness of breath, fatigue, and lowered resistance to infection. At Cleveland Metropolitan Hospital, John D. Hines concluded that "possibly 2% to 3% of subjects on the megadose regimen of ascorbic acid may well be at risk for ultimate development of vitamin B_{12} deficiency."

Hemolysis, or the destruction of red blood cells, can be induced by drugs or infection when individuals are deficient in the enzyme called erythrocyte glucose-6-phosphate dehydrogenase: G-6-PD for short. Dr. Martin H. Steinberg and two associates from the University of Mississippi School of Medicine reported on an individual with G-6-PD deficiency who developed intravascular hemolysis and acute kidney failure after being treated with large amounts of ascorbic acid. The patient, a sixty-eight-year-old black man, had been given 80 grams (80,000 mg) of ascorbic acid intravenously on each of two consecutive days.

Certainly caution and appropriate testing should be done before large doses of ascorbic acid are administered to individuals who might be susceptible to G-6-PD deficiency—American blacks, Sephardic Jews, and Orientals.

However, irrespective of the enzyme deficiency (which was assumed to be the basic cause of the man's death), it is clear that such a reaction would *not* occur from the oral ingestion of vitamin C. In fact, G. N. Schrauzer of the University of California in San Diego doubts death would have resulted from intravenous injection had sodium ascorbate—rather than free ascorbic acid—been used. He cites lower-animal experimental results to substantiate that contention.

To our knowledge, only two other reports—each limited to a single patient with sickle-cell disease—point to vitamin C's causing crises in individuals with deficient G-6-PD. It's hard to imagine that the three cases reported by Steinberg, by Herbert, and by Goldstein record the only G-6-PD patients who have been exposed to large quantities of vitamin C. Too, rare indeed is the individual who would take (or be given) 80,000 mg of ascorbic acid at a time—by mouth *or* by injection.

But back to B_{12} deficiency. What have other researchers found?

The Good News A group of scientists headed by Harold L. Newmark noted that the vitamin B_{12} content of the meals analyzed by Herbert and Jacob was much lower than the amount calculated from published values. After incubating meals of "modest" and "high" vitamin B_{12} content with increasing levels of vitamin C, the Newmark group reported *no* significant effect. They explain these differences as arising from their use of a more efficient B_{12} extraction and assay method. Thus, when standardized and official extraction methods are used, the Herbert and Jacob results appear to be impossible to duplicate.

Marcus and two co-workers from the Lincoln Medical and

Mental Health Center in the Bronx, New York, reported in vivo work that seems to preclude a B_{12} deficiency's developing from taking C. They state that B_{12} "is completely unaffected at body temperature by as much as 10 mg/ml of ascorbic acid"—a judgment echoed in an intensive study conducted by H. P. C. Hogenkamp at the University of Minnesota's Department of Biochemistry.

Similar conclusions were drawn in the *Journal of the American Medical Association* by an investigative team from the Saint Louis University Group Hospitals and Veterans Administration Hospital. In these hospitals it is routine procedure for all spinal-cord-injury patients to receive 4 grams (4000 mg) of C per day to enhance urinary acidity—thereby reducing such patients' high risk of urinary-tract infection. Over an eleven-month period of careful scrutiny, serum B_{12} levels remained normal to high.

At the Medical College of Wisconsin, Jerome J. DeCosse and some colleagues measured B_{12} blood levels in subjects being given 1 gram of ascorbic acid three times a day—that is, 3000 mg daily —over a period of thirteen months. They found *no* evidence of B_{12} destruction.

Our conclusion? Once again, some uncommon metabolic disorders may alter a person's chemistry so that the synthesis of certain co-enzymes could be interfered with, or so that normal biochemical sequences could be interrupted. But, by and large, there is *not* a connection between vitamin C and the destruction of vitamin B_{12}. If someone tells you otherwise, have him or her check the studies we've mentioned.

DIAGNOSTIC TESTS

Blood

Some doctors have declared that vitamin C in the blood interferes with the measurement of glucose. However, there are, as far as we can determine, no definitive reports that demonstrate this claim. On the contrary, reports indicate that vitamin C does *not* interfere with measurement of glucose in the blood. A few examples follow.

At the Jefferson Medical Center in Philadelphia, Sheila Katz and Thomas DiSilvio measured glucose in blood serum as they varied the concentration of ascorbic acid from 0.25 to 16.0 mg percent. Because vitamin C is so rapidly excreted in urine, it is unlikely that serum values of 16 mg percent could ever occur. In fact, Herbert E. Spiegel and Evelyn Pinili contend that a blood ascorbic acid above 2.5 mg percent simply can't occur from ingesting vitamin C and "must be judged as resulting from unphysiological artefacts." It was only at this extreme of 16 mg percent that there was a significant elevation of the average glucose value above the control sample. Even then, the increase amounted only to 4.2 mg percent. The researchers conclusion: "The automatic analyzer method for serum glucose may be used in the presence of elevated serum ascorbic acid levels without adversely affecting the diagnostic value of the test."

Another false alarm concerns diabetes, that is, that high levels of C might cause diabetes because they sometimes may cause slight increases in serum glucose values. According to scientists from the Departments of Medicine and Pathology, Pritzker School of Medicine and the Division of Biological Sciences at the University of Chicago: not so! Rubenstein and co-workers showed that intravenously administered doses of 1 and 2 grams of C given every three hours do not affect normal subjects' tolerance for glucose. Nor do they significantly alter fasting plasma glucose levels or affect serum insulin, glucagon, or growth-hormone levels. And these findings held despite a three- to eightfold rise in plasma ascorbic-acid concentration. The researchers concluded that "the acute administration of large doses of ascorbic acid has minimal effects on glucose tolerance in nondiabetic individuals."

As a matter of fact, as we outlined in Chapter 9, ascorbic acid appears to be *therapeutic* in diabetes.

Writing from Munich, Germany, Dr. Heinz W. Prauer cites the work of Mehnert, Forster, and Funke as additional evidence that high C intake will not impair glucose tolerance. Prauer gave 1500-mg doses for six weeks to healthy subjects and for five days to diabetics. "In healthy subjects no change of glucose tolerance was found during the period of observation, nor was there evidence of appreciable quantities of glucose or other reducing substances in the urine. In diabetic subjects no deterioration of the metabolic situation was noticed."

Finally, responding to a warning by M. H. Briggs and colleagues that bringing blood vitamin C levels to high levels might interfere with estimating serum bilirubin, S. R. V. Nobile and colleagues at the Vitamin Laboratories of Roche Products in New South Wales reported—in highly scientific language we're trying to simplify here—that the serum concentrations of vitamin C used by the Briggs group simply do not occur in nature.

It seems fairly obvious, however, that if you are going to test for blood glucose levels, you will not previously administer a high intravenous dose of C.

Stool

Each year, more than 30 million tests are given to see if there is blood in the stool, which might indicate bowel disease and many other disorders. Large doses of vitamin C can cause false-negative results; that is, they may obscure detection of the blood. Two chemically similar compounds, reductone and reductic acid, have the same effect. They are derived from refined sugar under conditions such as those found in the duodenum (the first part of the small intestine). Since the average American eats 140 pounds of refined sugar each year, it could be that reductone and reductic acid are the culprits.

Alas, no one seems to have investigated these chemicals as they might work to jinx the accuracy of tests for occult (hidden) blood in the stool. But vitamin C *has* been investigated. It is definitely known to influence false-negative results in stool tests. It takes little medical sophistication to guess the answer: temporarily desist!

At the National Institutes of Health, Russell M. Jaffe and coworkers reported on a woman known to have blood in her stools but who showed negative results in testing. When she agreed to temporarily stop taking her 1- to 2-gram daily dose of vitamin C, stool tests were positive within seventy-two hours. Jaffe and his colleagues concluded that 55 mg of C per day in the feces can inhibit the most commonly used blood tests. This is the amount of unabsorbed, fecally excreted ascorbic acid that could be expected from a daily intake of more than 750 mg of C. Restriction of supplementation for seventy-two hours before stool blood testing allows sufficient time for the digestive tract to clear itself of unabsorbed C.

Newer tests in which vitamin C in the stool cannot affect the search for blood have been developed by Jaffe and Zierdt and by a group at the University of Louisville School of Medicine headed by George H. Barrows.

Urine

It's rather widely claimed that vitamin C can cause inaccurate readings of urinary glucose measurements. This could be of special importance to diabetics who test their own urine for "sugar" and then adjust their treatment accordingly.

Most laboratories screen urine specimens with the glucose oxidase enzyme strip test and then quantitate positive results with a copper reduction test. Enzyme strip tests such as Labstix (Ames) and Tes-Tape (Lilly) are sensitive and will allow detection of glucose in as low a concentration as 10 mg percent or less—but they're not highly accurate for measuring the exact quantity.

From the Department of Pathology of the University of California at Irvine and the Orange County Medical Center in Orange, California, a research group led by James S. Mayson reported on the subject. They found that ascorbic acid may partially inhibit these strip tests when it is present in urine in a concentration as low as 10 mg percent. When ascorbic acid was added to urine in vitro (in the test tube), a concentration of 25 mg percent completely shut off the glucose-oxidase reaction. The same research team also demonstrated that adding ascorbic acid to urine could cause a false-positive reaction to the copper reduction glucose test (Clinitest by Ames). ("False-positive" means that a test shows something when it's not really there.) The higher the concentration of C, the worse the effect noted.

But how about human beings, rather than test tubes? Milap C. Nahata and Don C. McLeod, from the College of Pharmacy, Ohio State University in Columbus and the State University of New York at Buffalo, studied ten normal, nondiabetic male volunteers who were given 4 and 6 grams (4000 and 6000 mg) of ascorbic acid daily, divided into four or five doses. Each subject's urine was tested thirty-six times for glucose—nine times on each of the four dosage regimens. A total of 360 glucose-detection tests with the copper reduction method (Clinitest) were made and not one urine sample gave a positive reaction. Nahata and McLeod say: "It is possible that oral doses of ascorbic acid higher than 6 g. daily would result in a false-positive reading [but] this is unlikely, due to the decreased absorption with larger doses."

Jaffe's group (cited earlier) warns that ascorbic acid can inhibit detection of blood in the urine when chemical screening tests such as Multistix (Ames) are used. They also say that at higher levels it will interfere with microscopic analysis. For example, at 35 mg percent ascorbic acid, more than twenty erythrocytes per high-power field—a system of measuring red blood cells in urine with a microscope—were undetectable.

Just as we noted under the section describing stool tests for blood, the answer is simple: withhold C supplementation and C-rich foods (primarily citrus fruit or juice) for forty-eight to seventy-two hours before the testing is done.

What to Know and What to Do

The bottom line on vitamin C and diagnostic testing is that many of the warnings are without factual support.

But we've seen that some false-negative and some false-positive reactions have been found, and it's entirely possible that future research will uncover other effects.

If vitamin C must be withheld prior to certain diagnostic tests, it is certainly not alone! More than two dozen commonly used medications must be withdrawn before testing because they could influence results. Quite apart from pills, one may be instructed to abstain from many foods and liquids—or, in some cases, to abstain from food altogether! To prevent false-positive results in one stool-blood test, people are asked to refrain from eating meat, fish, poultry, and peroxidase-rich vegetables such as green beans and radishes for seventy-two hours before the test is performed.

For any type of biological testing, withdrawal of non-life-sustaining medicines and nutrients for several days before the test is a practical procedure. It should not suggest that any of these substances, including vitamin C, are necessarily harmful.

DIARRHEA AND DIGESTION

As the careful reader of this book knows by now, many clinicians and researchers have discussed C's connection to diarrhea. In fact, some doctors use the beginning of diarrhea as a gauge for backing off from the high doses initially needed to combat physical or mental stress. They do maintain, however, that continuing a mild-diarrhea dosage usually leads to digestive adaptation so that intestinal tolerance may increase to accommodate up to 30 and 40 grams per day.

What happens, quite simply, is that, when ingested vitamin C exceeds the digestive tract's ability to absorb it, some of the unabsorbed C enters the colon and causes a looseness of the bowels. The amount required to reach this stage may range from 3 to 10 grams per day. Substituting sodium ascorbate for all or part of the ascorbic acid dose can improve tolerance in those who react adversely; it can also minimize any complaints of too much gas.

On the other side of the coin, the elimination habits of millions of people could be significantly improved by vitamin C's laxative action. An increase from one to two (or even three) eliminations daily with added C and dietary fiber would be a plus factor in maintaining good bowel health.

As for the stomach, ascorbic acid will not lead to ulcers. In fact, if ulcers are present, this weak acid enhances healing.

Finally, according to S. Lewin of the North East London Polytechnic, 3 grams of vitamin C in the form of sodium ascorbate is about equal in alkalinity to 1.5 grams of sodium bicarbonate. This knowledge could be valuable to people who require an antacid reaction but who may experience stomach upset if they take an alkali such as soda.

INFERTILITY

Back in the first half of the 1970s, M. H. Briggs (Alfred Hospital's Department of Biochemistry in Victoria, Australia) stated: "I should like to propose a hypothesis [that] women taking excess vitamin C may have reduced fertility." Doctor Briggs's hypothesis followed observations that the reported reduction in cold symptoms may be caused by vitamin C's mucolytic (mucus-dissolving) action in the respiratory tract. He proposed that C may have a similar action on mucus of the uterine cervix, which could impair sperm penetration and prevent conception. His initial report was based on two presumably healthy young women who failed to conceive when they were taking 2 to 5 grams of ascorbic acid each day, but who did become pregnant after they stopped the supplementation. Briggs added six more such cases and asserted that these women's experiences "raise the suspicion that regular daily doses of ascorbic acid of two grams or more may reduce fertility in some individuals."

Dr. Abram Hoffer disagrees. For more than twenty years he has been giving large (2 to 10 grams per day) doses of ascorbic acid to more than 3000 women and reports no lowering of fertility. On the contrary, in what he describes as a "ten minute search" through his files, Hoffer produced the histories of four women who had conceived while they were taking 2 or 3 grams of C per day.

At Gunma University's School of Medicine in Maebashi, Japan, Masao Igarashi used ascorbic acid in oral doses of 400 mg to induce ovulation in a group of women in whom the fertility drug, clomiphene, had not worked. One in five subsequently became pregnant.

Cedric Wilson and H. S. Loh of the Department of Pharmacology at the University of Dublin in Ireland experimented with higher doses—500 to 2000 mg daily—in three women unable to conceive. One subject showed the normal (note: *normal*) preovulatory peak in urinary excretion of ascorbic acid and she then conceived after artificial insemination.

Could It Be True?

In Chapter 16, under the subheading "Fertility," we describe some work (including Dr. Igarashi's) that shows vitamin C's potential in increasing fertility.

If things were the other way around—that is, if vitamin C tended to make women *and men* infertile—any search for the safest and cheapest contraceptive method would immediately end! But as things are, with thousands of doctors prescribing C and millions of people taking it in doses of 2000 mg or more, the medical literature ought to be filled with reports substantiating Dr. Briggs's hypothesis!

KIDNEY STONES

Calcium Oxalate

No one questions that some portion of ingested vitamin C is metabolized to oxalate. Calcium oxalate can appear in the urine in the form of crystals and it is a major component of calculi or "stones."

However, many authorities believe that the amount is far too insignificant to implicate vitamin C. Steven R. Tannenbaum, Professor of Food Chemistry at MIT, says that "the conception that excess amounts of ascorbic acid lead to the formation of oxalic acid in the urine is simply not correct." This assessment was borne out in an experiment Lamden and Chrystowski performed when they measured oxalate excretion and discovered that increased C intake had no significant effect.

On the other hand are reports by M. H. Briggs of the Australian hospital mentioned earlier. Taking as his starting point a personal communication concerning a man who passed a urinary oxalate stone after taking 2 grams of ascorbic acid each day for two weeks, Briggs and his co-workers found a presumably healthy twenty-one-year-old man whose urinary oxalate rose from 58 mg to 478 and 622 mg, respectively, after four and seven days of taking 1 gram of C four times a day.

But Briggs himself—commenting on the first case—states that "development of a stone in such a short period suggests that this man may be one of the occasional individuals who converts high doses of vitamin C to urinary oxalate with efficiency." The reader should note the word *occasional* and also remember that the report originated from a personal communication that omits data about other factors that may have influenced stone development.

At the Wood Veterans Administration Hospital and Medical College of Wisconsin, Roth and Breitenfield reported on a young man whose physical examination, microscopic urinalysis, intravenous pyelogram, and family history were all negative for kidney disease. Urine levels were normal for calcium, phosphorus, and uric acid, but urinary oxalate was high. He was asked to stop taking the 1000 mg of ascorbic acid he'd been taking to prevent colds, and the oxalate excretion dropped.

It's important to note, we think, that one "postexperimental" level (62 mg/24 hours) was only 14 mg lower than one of the measurements (76 mg/24 hours) taken when the young man was still taking 1 gram of C daily. Also, the report omits any information about the subject's dietary oxalate intake (Barness says it accounts for 50 percent of oxalic acid excreted) or other factors that may play a role in stone formation.

At the Mayo Clinic, Lynwood H. Smith reported favorable results with five patients whose oxalate excretion decreased when they stopped taking vitamin C. But each patient had given a history of stones *before* they had begun taking C.

The fourth and last "bad" report we've been able to uncover comes from Victor Herbert, Professor and Vice-Chairman of Medicine at the State University of New York, Downstate Medical Center. Dr. Herbert says that some people—"possibly about one out of fifteen"—"have a congenital defect whereby they can't get ascorbate past the oxalic acid state readily, and those people will have an increased susceptibility to oxalate kidney stones." As a case in point, he describes having addressed medical students at Columbia University and discovering that "one of the medical students had just had an attack of renal colic due to a kidney stone after seven weeks of following his mother's advice to take a gram of C each morning prior to breakfast." Here, we decline comment!

The Good News   We've already given some reasons why we believe one need not be unduly worried about C's possible contribution to calcium-oxalate kidney stones—except in the rarest of instances. The fact is, the *reverse* is probably true: that is, ascorbic acid may *prevent* stone formation. Here's how:

1. Multigram doses of ascorbic acid increase the substance's presence in the urine. This gives rise to more acidic urine. Acid urine reduces the union of calcium and oxalate.
2. Vitamin C in the urine tends to bind calcium and decrease its free form. This means less chance of calcium's separating out as calcium oxalate.
3. Spillage of vitamin C into the urine enhances diuresis—that is, you urinate oftener. Since stone formation requires static conditions, increasing urine flow could inhibit the development of calculi.

There are other participants in oxalate metabolism. In an extensive review of the scientific literature, Hagler and Herman cite eleven interrelated nutritional factors.

1. High oxalate consumption
2. Low calcium intake (see Smith and colleagues)
3. Low magnesium intake (see Gershoff and Prien)
4. Ingestion of the common food preservative called EDTA
5. Primary or secondary deficiency of vitamin B_6 (see Gershoff and Prien)
6. High dietary tryptophan
7. Primary or secondary deficiency of vitamin B_1
8. High blood levels of vitamin D
9. High sucrose intake (see Thom and colleagues)
10. Inadequate water intake
11. Persistently acid urine

It appears that oxalate excretion may actually be minor as a cause of stones. Many individuals with normal oxalate excretion have calcium-oxalate urinary stones, while others without stones excrete large amounts of oxalate. As Tiselius found, the situation is just about the same:

SUBJECTS	DAILY MG OF OXALIC ACID EXCRETED
Normals	28.0
Stone patients	27.5

In addition to what's noted above—and readers who are interested in the details of the particular studies cited with the numbered list are urged to look them up in a university or college library—other stone contributors appear to be at work. For instance, soft water may not be so desirable as laundry-burdened or tub-scrubbing persons might think. The hospitalization rates for kidney stones are highest in areas where the mineral content of water is less than 50 parts per million. According to Churchill and co-workers, zinc, strontium, manganese, and cadmium restrain the renal calcification process.

High Oxalate Consumption Since this is number one in Hagler and Herman's list, concerned readers might want to be careful not to overload on high-oxalate foods. A serving of canned spinach contains about 350 mg of oxalic acid and each 12 ounces of cola or beer contains from 4 to 10 mg.

Careless eating (and drinking) could allow one easily to exceed the normal urinary oxalate excretion rate, which ranges anywhere from 38 to 100 mg in twenty-four hours.

Here is a list of *high-oxalate foods:*

beans	kale
beets	oranges
berries (especially blackberries,	parsley
currants, raspberries, and	peppers
strawberries)	plums
carrots	rhubarb

celery

coffee and cocoa (especially
  instant)

cucumbers

dandelion leaves

endive

spinach

sweet potatoes

tea

turnip tops

Comment Since all disease is caused by multiple interrelating factors, it seems absurd to think that the intake of vitamin C alone causes calcium-oxalate kidney stones. The evidence just presented indicates that many other factors come into play, and probably any one of them is more intimately involved than ascorbic acid. Naturally the rare person who, because of impaired metabolism, readily converts vitamin C into oxalic acid is in a high-risk category. But such an individual is usually aware of his or her defective chemistry to begin with.

Uric Acid

Stein and co-workers studied the effect ascorbic-acid supplementation may have on attacks of gouty arthritis and the formation of uric-acid stones in the urinary tract. They report a "cutoff point" of 4 grams: less did not significantly increase the excretion of uric acid, 4 grams did. However, the blood-serum level of uric acid remained constant. With higher doses (8 grams), the serum uric-acid level decreased by 1.2 to 3.1 mg percent as a result of urinary excretion. The researchers suggest that "vitamin C could invalidate studies involving the measurement of uric acid and obscure the diagnosis of gout." The solution seems simple: withhold supplementation before biochemical testing, as we detailed earlier in this chapter.

The same investigators also warn that vitamin C could "precipitate attacks of gouty arthritis or renal calculi in predisposed persons." However, as far as we've been able to determine, there is not a single published report that attests to this effect. Indeed, a new *treatment* for gout is suggested by the fact that megadoses of ascorbic acid cause a lowering of serum-uric-acid level because of increased urinary excretion!

REBOUND SCURVY

Although we've not been able to uncover any scientific evidence to support Gerhard N. Schrauzer's claim, the University of California at San Diego chemistry professor believes that suddenly stopping large doses of vitamin C can lead to attacks of scurvy. Together with Dr. William J. Rhead of UCSD's School of Medicine, Schrauzer ascribes the process to "enzyme induction." The contention? Humans adapt to C megadoses and activate enzymes that break down the excess C into other useful substances. Rhead and Schrauzer maintain that, when C intake is abruptly halted, this hyperactivity of enzymes drives the body's vitamin C content down to deficiency levels, leading to "rebound scurvy."

Only anecdotal material about several single cases is given to illustrate the phenomenon Rhead and Schrauzer describe. The experimental basis for the concept of rebound scurvy appears to be findings such as those presented by Edward Norkus and Pedro Rosso of the College of Physicians and Surgeons at Columbia University. They reported that offspring from guinea pigs receiving high levels of ascorbic acid during pregnancy develop scurvy sooner than do those born of animals receiving standard levels of this vitamin. They suggest that an increased rate of catabolism (breakdown) of vitamin C accounts for the offsprings' higher ascorbic-acid requirement. There seems to have been no experimental work among human beings—although we're aware of a report out of Halifax, Nova Scotia, concerning scurvy in two babies whose mothers consumed supplemental vitamin C.

But the children's condition was not adequately described. Could it have reflected a vitamin K deficiency rather than scurvy? And could this happen only in Halifax? With thousands and thousands of pregnant women taking vitamin C, would this "scurvy" not be a common observation?

We probably need not pose the questions, for several researchers have succeeded in disproving the rebound-scurvy/enzyme-induction hypothesis. At a research laboratory in Basel, Switzerland, a team headed by D. Hornig administered massive doses of ascorbic acid to guinea pigs, over a long period of time. They report that results "disprove the hypothesis that the regular ingestion of large doses of ascorbic acid may lead to systemic conditioning, i.e., accelerated ascorbic acid metabolism or excretion due to a possible induction of the participating enzymes." The team also cites similar conclusions reached in 1964 by Kieckebusch.

As for the alleged pregnancy connection, massive doses of C were administered to lower animals (guinea pigs, rats, mice, and hamsters) in experiments conducted by F. R. Alleva and colleagues at the Food and Drug Administration and by H. Frohberg at a toxicology institute in Germany. There were no adverse effects whatsoever in the adults or in the offspring. In fact, in the first-mentioned study there was a significant reduction in the number of stillbirths and an increase in the average weight of live pups in the C-treated group as compared with controls. It's also worth noting that in the German study doses ranged as high as 1000 mg per kg per day. In human terms, this is equivalent to a 130-pound woman's taking approximately 59,000 mg of vitamin C each day!

Finally, as far as a case report by Siegel and two colleagues goes, we find it difficult to accept their diagnosis of "conditioned oral scurvy" in a forty-nine-year-old man under their dental treatment. They believe that his bleeding mouth sores occurred as a rebound phenomenon when and because he stopped taking his customary 1 gram of ascorbic acid daily. Two major points seem to contradict their conclusion. First, the evidence presented could quite validly suggest that the patient needs a daily gram of C to maintain oral health. Second, the diagnosis was based purely on a nutritional history; no laboratory determinations of vitamin C levels were made.

Although there may be a decrease in the blood level of C for a week or two when megadoses are reduced to the RDA level, it has not been shown to pose a health hazard. Nonetheless, to be on the safe side, it may be wise to decrease supplementation gradually over a week or two rather than suddenly.

THROMBOSIS

D. F. Horrobin from the Department of Physiology of the Medical School at Newcastle-Upon-Tyne in England published a self-report concerning deep-vein thrombosis (a "thrombus" is a clot in a vessel). He believed it was induced by taking 3000 mg of vitamin C for a cold. Horrobin admits, however, that "the diagnosis was not confirmed by sophisticated techniques" and that the condition "resolved spontaneously over the next six days," a rather unusual course for thrombosis to follow.

The thrombus threat is probably another myth that can be laid to rest, particularly in view of a study performed in Basel, Switzerland, by Alfred B. Hanck, a scientist with Hoffmann-La Roche. Subjects were eleven healthy men and women, twenty-five to forty-five years of age, with no history of abnormal blood clotting. After a three-week trial of 4-gram daily doses of ascorbic acid, Hanck found no significant effect on the coagulation of blood.

SUMMING UP

High doses of vitamin C may affect the accuracy of certain diagnostic tests. But so can many other substances, which is why test-bound individuals are often asked to refrain from taking specific foods, liquids, and medications. It's the same with C. Simply temporarily suspend your supplementation.

Large doses of vitamin C do tend to cause diarrhea. One has a couple of options: back off to a lower dosage, or "hang in there" until the intestinal tract adapts. For many people, vitamin C's laxative effect may bring welcome relief.

It's also clear that caution should be exercised when professionals contemplate intravenous injection of large ascorbic-acid doses in individuals susceptible to G-6-PD deficiency.

As for the other grim tales—ranging from B_{12} deficiency to kidney stones—let us simply say that the reports of C's evils are *greatly* exaggerated! Indeed, in the absence of scientific evidence more convincing than the negative studies we're aware of and have mentioned in this chapter, we are inclined to think C is innocent of the bad effects ascribed to it. As a matter of fact, in at least two cases—diabetes and infertility—ascorbic acid is known to help, not hinder.

20
You Can't Live by C Alone

The message of this book is simple: with too little vitamin C, you'll be in poor health; if it is absent, you'll die. This is not some capricious notion. It is a hard-core fact, documented by almost countless scientific studies—many of which we've described in the preceding chapters.

But can one subsist on C alone? Of course not. There are more than forty essential nutrients; without any one of them, we'd eventually die. Each nutrient is linked to all the others, and they all act in an interrelated fashion. Exactly *how* this occurs is quite a complex matter indeed. But some insight may be gained by reading what Drs. Harte and Chow have to say in the classic nutrition textbook *Modern Nutrition in Health and Disease:*

> In the first edition of this book a comprehensive, critical review of relevant literature to 1953 included well over 200 references on the various facets of the problem of dietary interrelationships. Since then additional reports have appeared to further elucidate such dietary inter-relationships. Perhaps the most striking impression received from evaluation of the literature is that hardly any study undertaken with any pair of nutrients has failed to show a significant interaction in terms of some nutritional or biochemical criterion. This is not surprising, though, since each step of the chain of reactions through which a nutrient goes as it follows an appropriate metabolic pathway is mediated by at least one enzyme system, and the functioning of every enzyme system calls for the combined action of an apoenzyme (made up for the most part of amino acids) and a coenzyme (which usually includes a vitamin and/or a mineral element). However, the breadth of the experimental interrelationships brought out by these various studies underlines the statement that "the recognition of the large num-

ber of them re-emphasizes the basic soundness of the principle of maintaining variety in food in order to provide the most nourishing diet.

Thus, the biologic activity of carbohydrates, proteins, fats, vitamins, and minerals is so interdependent that an imbalance of any
one of them will probably affect most of the others. That's why a
variety of foods is necessary to provide appropriate amounts of
essential nutrients. For example, let's review vitamin C's connection to preventing or correcting iron-deficiency anemia by enhancing the absorption of iron present in foods we eat. C's effect
is directly proportional to the amount of the vitamin present at
mealtime, over a range of 25 to 1000 mg. Iron absorption from
food was increased from 1.65- to 9.57-fold. But the vitamin C and
the iron must be taken at the same time. Breakfast-time orange
juice or a C supplement won't influence iron uptake from later
meals or snacks. But daily iron absorption will more than double
when one's daily C intake is divided equally over three meals
rather than being taken at one meal only.

Even iron-deficient people who take iron supplements may not
attain good levels without the help of C. Sean Lynch, Associate
Professor of Hematology at the University of Kansas, and some
colleagues discovered that when patients take 100 mg of vitamin
C along with meat meals, they absorbed 40 percent more iron.
With vegetarian meals, the same amount of C doubled and even
tripled iron absorption. (This occurred because iron from meat,
fish, or poultry is more readily absorbed, so C's effect on vegetable meals would be expected to be stronger.) The Lynch team
found that just 25 mg of vitamin C would turn from 30 to 90
grams of meat, fish, or poultry into a high-iron category.

YOU AND YOUR SHOPPING CART

As we've already pointed out, it seems that food processors' advertising budgets are inversely related to a product's nutritional
value: the more worthless the food, the more expensive and elaborate the print ad or TV commercial. Michael Jacobson, Director
of the Center for Science in the Public Interest, takes an especially

dim view of this situation. He feels that major food marketers are cunning adversaries dedicated to profit rather than public health, and he says consumers should be on the lookout for companies' devious ways.

In fact, Dr. Jacobson is responsible for the following quiz, which will help you to assess your nutritional awareness. Circle either *A* or *B* as your answer to each question.

1. A number of food additives have been linked to detrimental health effects. If you were trying to avoid the two worst additives, you would read labels carefully to steer away from products containing (A) Polysorbate-60 and EDTA; (B) sugar and artificial coloring.
2. Fiber or roughage is removed from wheat and rice when they are processed. Since fiber does not contain any vitamins or minerals, it is nutritionally worthless. (A) True; (B) False.
3. You are sure to increase the nutritional adequacy of your diet by carefully choosing foods labeled as having been "enriched" during manufacture. (A) True; (B) False.
4. All fruits are good and nutritious, but the one that contains the most vitamins per average serving is (A) a wedge of watermelon; (B) an apple.
5. A wise choice for a nutritious and healthy dessert is fruit-flavored gelatin. (A) True; (B) False.
6. The riboflavin (vitamin B_2) that is contained in milk is best protected against loss by (A) a waxed-paper carton; (B) a clear glass bottle.
7. Meat is an excellent source of protein. You are making a better nutritional buy when purchasing (A) choice or prime cuts of beef; (B) good or standard grades of beef.
8. If you were relying on carrots for your daily vitamin A supply, you would be wise to eat (A) raw young tender carrots; (B) steamed or boiled older mature carrots.

How do you think you did? Score yourself as described below:

Question 1.	(A) 1 point;	(B) 2 points
Question 2.	(A) 1 point;	(B) 2 points
Question 3.	(A) 1 point;	(B) 2 points
Question 4.	(A) 2 points;	(B) 1 point
Question 5.	(A) 1 point;	(B) 2 points
Question 6.	(A) 2 points;	(B) 1 point
Question 7.	(A) 1 point;	(B) 2 points
Question 8.	(A) 1 point;	(B) 2 points

If you scored a perfect 16, you're nutritionally sophisticated and ought to be able to return from grocery shopping in good shape. But it's no guarantee; it takes considerable will power to resist the slick commercials calculated to earn more profits from nutrient-depleted foods—for example, breakfast cereals stripped of vitamins, minerals, vegetable oils, protein, and fiber, but saturated with sugar.

Too, even the most natural-seeming foods may fool you. Astute quiz takers may have noticed Dr. Jacobson's trick question: Question 8. Carrots do not contain appreciable amounts of vitamin A until they mature. Then, what A they do contain is locked into the cells. Thus, carrots are one of only a few vegetables that provide more nutrition when they're cooked than when they're nibbled raw.

Some Cardinal Rules

Wary buyers who want to get the most for their money and also ensure good nutrition can help themselves by following two rules described below.

Avoid Food Additives The less you eat doctored foods, the less likely you'll need doctoring! Remember that the nutritional value of a food is inversely proportional to its shelf life. That means that the higher a food's nutritional value is—especially in vitamins, minerals, essential amino acids and essential fatty acids—the shorter is its shelf life. Depleted foods are so heavily doctored with various additives they'll last indefinitely on your shelves. But they will not provide needed nutrients.

Nourishing foods, on the other hand, do spoil quickly. But it's smart business—both economically and for your family's nutrition—to buy foods in their natural state and simply dump all those two thousand additives that include not only a variety of dubious chemicals but preservatives in the form of salt and many kinds of sugar substances.

Take a look at the cost comparison made by Traub and Odland.

Cost per Serving of Ingredients for Home-Prepared and
Convenience Foods, July 1978–June 1979 (4-City Average)

PRODUCT	SERVING SIZE (OZ.)	HOME-PREPARED (CENTS)	CONVENIENCE FORMS (CENTS)
beef lasagna	9.8	57.7	112.6
beef meat loaf dinner	9.1	37.1	91.4
chicken a la king	5.7	27.8	47.4
fried chicken, batter-dipped	2.0	28.9	51.3
chicken salad, spread	2.5	23.0	46.4
pizza	8.3	37.8	73.2
cooked rice	3.4	2.8	4.2
broccoli au gratin	5.1	35.5	51.6
pork and beans	6.9	8.0	17.5
potatoes au gratin	4.5	10.7	35.8
boiled potatoes	4.0	4.1	14.3
hash-browned potatoes	3.9	5.8	13.5
potato patties	3.1	4.9	15.9
stuffed potatoes	5.6	14.1	31.1
scrambled eggs	4.1	14.8	28.6
angel food cake	1.7	6.3	15.5
pound cake	1.1	3.9	14.2
orange sherbet	3.2	6.2	13.4
yeast rolls	1.3	2.4	3.2

Take Three Meals—but Snack, Too Never try to get by on
less than three meals every day; breakfast, lunch, and dinner (or
supper). The first meal of the day is critically important: it gets
you ready for all the physical and mental challenges of the day.
You'll feel better and be able to maintain your true ideal weight a
lot more easily if you follow this guide: Eat breakfast like a king,
lunch like a prince, and dinner like a pauper.

You can also forget about the time-honored, popular, but false
belief that snacking between meals is automatically bad. In food-
frequency studies of adults, measures such as weight, blood pressure, blood sugar, and blood lipids were all reduced toward normal in those individuals who added nourishing midmorning or
afternoon snacks to their three-meals-per-day routine. Please note
that we said "nourishing"—that is, nutritional food, not junk

food. Confine your nibbling to items such as raw nuts and seeds, fresh fruit, raw vegetables, unsweetened fruit or vegetable juices, milk, yogurt, and cheese. These foods satisfy the body's need and also offer the bonus of helping to control your appetite when the next mealtime comes.

So—once you've chosen your snack foods wisely—nibble away! But never, never do it late in the evening, once you've eaten your evening meal. Late-night nibbling will affect your weight and other health parameters, and may contribute to a host of disorders.

THE OPTIMAL DIET

What we call "the optimal diet" was detailed in an earlier book authored by two of us. In essence, it is not a "diet" at all. It simply spells out optimal eating for optimal living. There are no menus to follow, no calories or carbohydrate grams to count, and no need to measure or weigh food portions or servings. All foods are simply categorized into one of three groups: (1) foods to eat liberally, (2) foods to eat sparingly, and (3) foods to avoid. Portions can and should be adjusted to suit an individual's appetite and goals. People who are underweight or overweight, as well as those with special nutritional requirements, find that the optimal diet helps readjust their metabolic balance; this can eliminate a host of food-related problems, disorders, or diseases. Above all, the optimal diet offers you a way to develop *rational eating habits* you can follow for the rest of your life.

Foods to Eat Liberally

It's especially important to eat foods that contain nutrients to enhance the body's defense system. These *resistance factors*—including protein, unrefined carbohydrates, essential fatty acids, and vitamins and minerals—are found in a variety of wholesome foods.

Because of vitamin C's "vanishing act," which we described in Chapter 2, processed foods should be avoided whenever possible.

Let your first choice be fresh foods; your second choice, frozen foods; your third, canned. However, vacuum-packed freeze-dried foods and dehydrated foods do retain enough nutrients to make them adequate for use in camping or hiking trips, or during seasons when fresh sources are scarce or when shortages exist because of strikes or crop failures. Vacuum-packed freeze-dried foods can be stored for long periods of time, even for several years.

Here's a list of foods to eat liberally.

beans (including dried beans)*
berries
brown rice*
cheese
corn*
eggs
fruit
meat
milk (preferably low-fat or skimmed)
nuts
peas (including dried peas)*
potatoes (Irish and sweet)*
poultry
seafood
seeds
vegetables
whole-corn meal*
whole grains (corn, oats, rice, rye, wheat)*
whole-grain breads*
whole-grain cereals*
whole-grain flours*
whole-grain pastas*

*Unrefined carbohydrates.

The Raw and the Cooked   Several of these food groups, such as fruits, berries, vegetables, nuts, and seeds, should be eaten *raw* each day with meals or snacks. When possible, it's best to eat the peelings of fruits and vegetables and the skins of nuts and seeds. These foods are ones that have largely been neglected in American diets, although the emergence of the salad bar has changed things for the better.

If fruits, berries, vegetables, nuts, and seeds *must* be cooked, you can preserve more nutritional value by adhering to the guidelines that follow, and, as we've suggested elsewhere in this book, you can always add some powdered ascorbic acid to bring back the C.

1. Don't boil the foods in water.
2. Bathe them in steam (away from the water that's generating the steam) by using a closed steamer or pressure cooker.
3. Cover or wrap these foods properly and cook them in a microwave oven.
4. Stir-fry any food for as short a time as possible in safflower or similar oil.

Unrefined Carbohydrates   These foods—asterisked in the list above—are comparatively inexpensive energy-producing sources. Unrefined carbohydrate-rich foods also provide fiber. Fiber is a regulator for both constipation and diarrhea, and it also aids in regulating appetite, blood sugar, blood lipids, and blood pressure. The correct amount of fiber in your diet will produce two (maybe three) bowel movements daily. This is desirable—even though to many constipated Americans it may seem like diarrhea.

An excellent source of fiber is unrefined wheat bran. This should not be confused with refined bran cereals in which what's added never makes up for what's been taken away.

Vegetarian Plans   For people who wish to abstain from meat, poultry, and seafood, adequate protein can be obtained from eggs, milk, and cheese when they're eaten with a proper combination of vegetables. Dr. Don Novey, a family practitioner in Carbondale, Illinois, gives this sensible advice for those who choose to be vegetarians. What one food may lack, another will supply in essential amino acids, the protein-building blocks. So simply match the following food pairs:

beans and seeds or nuts
beans and grains
dairy foods and beans

dairy foods and grains
dairy foods and seeds
grains and seeds or nuts

A Final Guideline   The real key is: use a wide variety of the
foods that should be eaten liberally. If you do this and follow
other suggestions outlined in this section, there's no need to be
concerned about the number or the size of servings.

Foods to Eat Sparingly

Here's a list of foods that should be eaten only on a limited basis.

animal fat
chocolate
cocoa
coffee
hydrogenated fats (margarine, peanut butter [in excess], shorten-
    ing, coffee whitener, and many convenience foods)
salt
soft drinks (especially the caffeinated varieties)
sugar
tea

Most people would benefit from reducing their intake of animal fat by trimming it from meat and by choosing leaner varieties of flesh, such as fish and chicken—and also by using low-fat or
skimmed milk.

Whenever fat *is* used for frying, seasoning, salad dressing, or as
part of a particular recipe, use a highly unsaturated vegetable oil
such as safflower, sunflower seed, or corn oil. You might want to
restrict your intake of the hydrogenated (chemically hardened)
fats that are listed above. The hydrogenation and refining of vegetable fat changes the molecular structure of fatty acids and produces a monster fat that human metabolism can't handle.

As for a spread for bread or potatoes, there's an excellent com-
promise between the saturated and the unsaturated. Blend two
softened sticks of unsalted creamery butter with 8 ounces of unrefined safflower oil. Then place the mixture in a covered container

and refrigerate. The result? A tasty and more healthy spread that has the consistency of tub margarine.

Almost everyone would benefit from a significant reduction in salt intake, especially people with high blood pressure or a tendency to retain fluid. The craving for salt is an acquired taste and one that's difficult to get over. But if you *gradually* reduce the salt you use, your taste buds will detect smaller quantities. Furthermore, all foods will come alive to your taste buds when they aren't laden with excess salt.

The same goes for sugar. Substituting honey may be a good idea, since it's twice as sweet as table sugar (so you use less) and is principally fructose—a form of sugar that is better tolerated (even by diabetics and hypoglycemics) than sucrose is.

Finally, there's the question of caffeine—coffee, tea, and a wide variety of soft drinks. Increasing evidence points to caffeine's linkage to impaired stress tolerance, hypoglycemia (low blood sugar), emotional disorders, birth defects, and cystic breast disease. If you insist on having coffee (or tea), drink it only with meals, and if you feel miserable drinking it unsweetened, use a low-calorie sweetener, but try to avoid using such a product in other foods.

Foods to Avoid

It seems fairly obvious that people should avoid eating or drinking things that increase the likelihood of poor health or disease. But it's also clear that many people aren't too sure just what these items are. Here is a partial list.

alcohol	graham crackers
artificial coloring agents	hot chocolate
artificial flavorings	ice cream
highly processed or refined	ice milk
grain foods (corn, oats,	lozenges
rice, rye, wheat)	milkshakes
sugar-high foods	mints
"athletic beverages"	pies
bran muffins	popsicles

cakes and icings
candy
candied sweet potatoes
    (or in syrup)
chocolate
chocolate milk
chocolate sauce
coffee cakes
cookies
cough drops
custards
dessert wines and cordials
doughnuts
frozen desserts
fruit drinks (canned
    or frozen)
fruit in syrup (canned
    or frozen)

puddings
punch drinks
sherbet
sweet pickles
sweet rolls
sweet syrups
sweetened applesauce (and
    other sweetened sauces)
sweetened breakfast cereals
sweetened breakfast
    drinks
sweetened soft drinks
sweetened yogurt

Keep in mind that this is only a partial list and that many other foods on your supermarket shelf may be excessively high in sugar content. Even if you studiously peruse a product's label, you can't always be sure. As most people know, ingredients are listed in descending order of quantity. But let's take an example. The word "sugar" itself may not be near the top of the list, but watch out for these terms: sucrose, invert sugar, turbinado sugar, brown sugar, dextrose, glucose, corn syrup, and corn sweeteners. When several of these terms appear on the same label, the food can be predominately sugar despite the fact that the word "sugar" may appear far from the top of the list.

With the possible exception of alcohol, sugar is the most potentially harmful of the foods to avoid eating. Sucrose can have some devastating effects on the body, as outlined below.

METABOLIC DEFECTS INDUCED BY DIETARY SUCROSE	DISORDERS INFLUENCED BY METABOLIC DEFECT
decreases action of sialin (a decay-inhibiting chemical in saliva)	dental caries (cavities, decay)
increases dental plaque	caries, periodontal disease
increases *Candida albicans*	oral and vaginal moniliasis
decreases phagocytosis	all infectious disorders
increases blood cholesterol	cardiovascular disease
increases bile cholesterol	gallstones
increases blood triglycerides	cardiovascular disease, gout, diabetes
increases platelet stickiness	cardiovascular disease
increases blood sugar	diabetes, cardiovascular disease, periodontal disease, gout, others
increases blood uric acid	gout, diabetes, cardiovascular disease
increases blood insulin	reactive hypoglycemia, diabetes, periodontal disease
increases body fat	overweight, diabetes, cardiovascular disease, gout, others
increases intestinal transit time	disorders of colon and rectum, varicose veins, hemorrhoids
increases urinary calcium excretion	urinary stones, osteoporosis (including tooth-supporting bone loss)
increases urine pH	urinary stones, genito-urinary infections
increases gastric acidity	indigestion, peptic ulcer
encourages malnutrition	all diseases
increases blood pressure	hypertension, cardiovascular diseases
increases tissue lactic acid during circulatory arrest	brain and CNS damage

The second large category of foods to avoid eating is those composed primarily of refined wheat flour or "white flour" as it's often called. In addition to items you might easily imagine—such as white breads, pancakes, rolls, muffins, hamburger buns, English muffins, biscuits, crackers, pretzels, and the usual (non-whole-grain) pastas—the group contains all of the sweetened baked products listed earlier.

And, while you're reading labels, don't be fooled by the phrase "enriched flour." Of the more than twenty vitamins, minerals, and essential amino acids removed as wheat is transformed into white flour, only four are added back. These are vitamin B_1, vitamin B_2, niacin, and iron. This is "enrichment"? It doesn't take a mathematical genius to see that -20 and $+4$ combine to make -16.

Another problem stems from preservatives. Under a heading called "The Nitrite Scene" in Chapter 10, we discussed the carcinogenic potential of the nitrites and nitrates present in bacon, ham, all kinds of presliced and packaged sandwich meats, corned beef, canned luncheon meats, salami, bologna, most frankfurters, liverwurst, smoked fish, and other processed meats and meat products. Here one has, at least, a fighting chance, for such products are appropriately labeled. Not so with most of the food colors, flavors, and preservatives. If you notice "sodium nitrate," "sodium nitrite," "artificial color," "artificial flavoring," or similar wording, try to avoid the food product.

WHY SUPPLEMENTS?

If you follow our optimal diet, will you get an adequate supply of all the essential nutrients, including vitamin C? Well, "adequate" probably, but "optimal," not a chance!

First of all, too much nutritional value is lost in the garden-to-gullet transit. Various processing techniques, plus transportation, storage, freezing, thawing, canning, cooking, and an almost inevitable time lapse between cooking and eating all combine to destroy nutrients in a way that's hard for even the most health-conscious individual to combat.

Readers of this book know that many factors can deplete their body stores of C. Increased nutritional requirements can be caused by individual biochemistry, psychological stress, surgical operations, physical trauma from accidents, many kinds of illnesses, lack of exercise, environmental pollution, the aging process, literally hundreds of medicines, and other factors too numerous to repeat here. Food alone—even our optimal diet!—cannot assure this hedge against nutrient depletion.

When you're choosing a dietary supplement, it's wise to remember that it should provide all the essential vitamins and minerals plus the mistakenly named *non*essential elements. A supplement should be taken before or during each of your three meals—but certainly no less than twice daily. This will ensure that all of the more than forty nutrients are present at the same time in the digestive tract—a situation that must be maintained for optimal growth, maintenance, and any needed repair of the body's cells, tissues, organs, and systems.

What is a good vitamin-mineral supplement? We feel that a good one will provide daily dosages of nutrients approximating the quantities listed below.

Vitamin A	12,500	to	25,000	IU
Vitamin D	500	to	1,000	IU
Vitamin E (d alpha tocopherol)	300	to	600	IU
Vitamin C	750	to	1,500	mg
Bioflavonoid complex	400	to	800	mg
Rutin	50	to	100	mg
Hesperidin complex	50	to	100	mg
Folic acid	0.4	to	0.8	mg
Vitamin B_1 (thiamine)	12.5	to	25	mg
Vitamin B_2 (riboflavin)	12.5	to	25	mg
Niacin	50	to	100	mg
Vitamin B_6 (pyridoxine)	12.5	to	25	mg
Vitamin B_{12}	125	to	250	mcg
Biotin	75	to	150	mcg
Choline	100	to	200	mg
Inositol	100	to	200	mg
Pantothenic acid	100	to	200	mg
PABA	50	to	100	mg
Calcium	350	to	700	mg
Phosphorus	100	to	200	mg
Magnesium	175	to	350	mg
Zinc	25	to	50	mg
Potassium	90	to	180	mg
Iodine	0.125	to	0.250	mg
Iron	15	to	30	mg
Copper	0.1	to	0.2	mg
Manganese	5	to	10	mg
Selenium	50	to	100	mcg
Chromium	50	to	100	mcg
Molybdenum	50	to	100	mcg

If by chance the optimal diet causes some indigestion at first, or if you already suffer from this malady, digestive supplements may be helpful. The two most likely to relieve indigestion of the non-acidic variety are digestive enzymes and hydrochloric acid. You can very simply test your possible need for a hydrochloric-acid supplement. One or two teaspoons of vinegar with each meal will let you know in a day or so. If it relieves the indigestion, consult a doctor about taking hydrochloric acid. If the vinegar worsens your indigestion, or does not relieve it, stop using it.

We also invite you—as we've done throughout this book—to consult with a nutrition-oriented health professional who can further advise you on appropriate supplementation, as well as general dietary practices. But, whether you do it with professional help or on your own, *do it:* improve your nutrition and watch your health improve.

Bibliography

1. Why C?

Cooke, W. L., and Milligan, R. S. Recurrent Hemoperitoneum Reversed by Ascorbic Acid. *Journal of the American Medical Association* 237: 13, 1358–1359, 28 March 1977.

Maxwell, R. *Health Care: The Growing Dilemma.* 1975. New York, McKinsey and Company.

May, J. M. The Ecology of Human Disease. *Annals of the New York Academy of Sciences* 84:17, 789–794, December 1960.

Pauling, L. *Vitamin C, The Common Cold and the Flu.* 1976. San Francisco, W. H. Freeman and Company.

2. Vitamin C's "Vanishing Act"

Augustin, J. Variations in the Nutritional Composition of Fresh Potatoes. *Journal of Food Science* 40:6, 1295–1299, November/December 1975.

Bender, A. E. The Fate of Vitamins in Food Processing Operations. In Stein, M. *Vitamins.* 1971. University of Nottingham Seminar. London, Churchill Livingstone.

Briggs, M., and Briggs, M. Vitamin C Requirements and Oral Contraceptives. *Nature* 238:5362, 277, 4 August 1972.

Bring, S. V., Grassl, C., Hofstrand, J. T., and Willard, M. J. Total Ascorbic Acid in Potatoes. *Journal of the American Dietetic Association* 42:4, 320–324, April 1963.

Bring, S. V., and Raab, F. P. Total Ascorbic Acid in Potatoes. *Journal of the American Dietetic Association* 45:2, 149-152, August 1964.

Cain, R. F. Technology of Fortification of Foods. Paper presented at a workshop sponsored by the Food Protection Committee, National Academy of Sciences, 1975.

Cheraskin, E., and Ringsdorf, W. M., Jr. Vitamin C State in a Dental School Patient Population. *Journal of the Southern California State Dental Association* 32:10, 375–378, October 1964.

Cheraskin, E., Ringsdorf, W. M., Jr., and Clark, J. W. *Diet and Disease.* 1977. New Canaan, Conn., Keats Publishing, Inc.

Citrus Sappers—Heat and Oxygen. *Science News* 117:13, 201, 29 March 1980.

Daniels, A. L., and Everson, G. J. Influence of Acetylsalicylic Acid (Aspirin) on Urinary Excretion of Ascorbic Acid. *Proceedings of the Society of Experimental Biology and Medicine* 35:1, 20–24, October 1936.

Dunbar, J. B., Cheraskin, E., Flynn, F. H., and Marley, J. F. The Intradermal Ascorbic Acid Test: Part IV. A Study of Tolerance Testing in Sixteen Dental Students. *Journal of Dental Medicine* 14:3, 131–155, July 1959.

Eddy, T. P. The Problem of Retaining Vitamins in Hospital Food. In Exton-Smith, A. N., and Scott, D. L. *Vitamins in the Elderly.* 1968. Bristol, John Wright and Sons, Ltd.

Fast Foods OK with Nutrition Know-How. *Medical Times* 107:7, 21–22, July 1979.

Fennema, O. Loss of Vitamins in Fresh and Frozen Foods. *Food Technology* 31:12, 32–35, December 1977.

Food Technology Altering Nutrition. *Nutrition Notes* 60:1, December 1973.

Fortification of Fruits, Vegetables Related to Losses During Processing. *Nutrition Notes* 68:7–8, April 1976.

Glew, G., Hill, M. A., and Millross, J. Vitamins: The Position Now in Large Scale Catering. In Stein, M. *Vitamins.* 1971. University of Nottingham Seminar. London, Churchill Livingstone.

Gortner, W. A. Food Technology in Australia. (United Fruit and Vegetable Association, Washington D.C.) *Nutrition Notes* 60:1, December 1973.

Government Researcher Reveals How Storing Produce Affects Nutrient Content. (An interview with John Krochta of the United States Department of Agriculture) *Nutrition Action* 6:3, 10–12, March 1979.

Harris, R. S. Influence of Culture on Man's Diet. *Archives of Environmental Health* 5:2, 144–152, August 1962.

Harris, R. S., and Karmas, E. *Nutritional Evaluation of Food Process-*

ing. Second Edition. 1975. Westport, Connecticut, The Avi Publishing Company, Inc.

Harris, R. S., and von Loesecke, H. *Nutritional Evaluation of Food Processing.* 1960. New York, Wiley.

Head, M. K. Nutrient Losses in Institutional Food Handling. *Journal of the American Dietetic Association* 65:4, 423–427, October 1974.

The Health Consequences of Smoking: A Public Health Service Review: 1967. PHS Publication No. 1696. United States Department of Health, Education, and Welfare.

The Health Consequences of Smoking: A 1969 Supplement to the 1967 Public Health Service Review. PHS Publication No. 1696-2. United States Department of Health, Education, and Welfare.

The Health Consequences of Smoking: A Report of the Surgeon General: 1972. DHEW Publication No. (HSM) 72-7516. United States Department of Health, Education, and Welfare.

Horwitt, M. K., Harvey, C. C., and Dahm, C. H. Relationship Between Levels of Blood Lipids, Vitamins C, A, and E, Serum Copper Compounds and Urinary Excretion of Tryptophan Metabolites Taking Oral Contraceptive Therapy. *American Journal of Clinical Nutrition* 28:4, 403–412, April 1975.

Hubbard, A. W. The American Diet Paradox. *Modern Medicine Topics* 23:12, December 1962.

Kahn, R. M. and Halliday, E. G. Ascorbic Acid Content of White Potatoes as Affected by Cooking and Standing on Steam Table. *Journal of the American Dietetic Association* 20:4, 220–222, April 1944.

Karel, M., and Heidelbaugh, N. D. Effects of Packaging on Nutrients. In Harris, R. S., and Karmas, E. *Nutritional Evaluation of Food Processing.* Second Edition. 1975. Westport, Conn., The Avi Publishing Company, Inc.

Lind, J. *A Treatise of the Scurvy.* First Edition. 1753. Edinburgh, Sands, Murray and Cochran.

Loh, H. S., Watters, K., and Wilson, C. W. M. The Effects of Aspirin on the Metabolic Availability of Ascorbic Acid in Human Beings. *Journal of Clinical Pharmacology* 13:11–12, 480–486, November/December 1973.

Marks, J. *A Guide to the Vitamins: Their Role in Health and Disease.* 1975. Lancaster, England, Medical and Technical Publishing Company.

McCormick, W. J. Ascorbic Acid: A Chemotherapeutic Agent. *Archives of Pediatrics* 69:4, 151–155, April 1952.

Morgan, A. F. *Nutritional Status, U.S.A.* 1959. Berkeley, California Agricultural Experiment Station, Bulletin 769.

Nicotine from Other Smokers. *Science News* 107, 15 February 1975.

Nonsmokers Affected by Tobacco Smoke. *Science News* 117:14, 221, 5 April 1980.

OCs—Update on Usage, Safety, and Side Effects. Population Reports: Oral Contraceptives. Series A, Number 5, January 1979. Population Information Program, Johns Hopkins University, Hampton House, 624 North Broadway, Baltimore, Maryland 21205.

Pantos, C. E., and Markakis, P. A Research Note: Ascorbic Acid Content of Artifically Ripened Tomatoes. *Journal of Food Science* 38:3, 550, March/April 1973.

Pelletier, O. Cigarette Smoking and Vitamin C. *Nutrition Today* 5:3, 12–15, Autumn 1970.

Prasad, A. S., Lei, K. Y., Oberleas, D., Moghissi, K. S., and Stryker, J. Effect of Oral Contraceptive Agents on Nutrients. II. Vitamins. *American Journal of Clinical Nutrition* 28:4, 385–391, April 1975.

Ringsdorf, W. M., Jr., and Cheraskin, E. Vitamin C and the Metabolism of Analgesic, Antipyretic, and Anti-Inflammatory Drugs: A Review. *Alabama Journal of Medical Sciences* 16:3, 217–220, July 1979.

Rivers, J. M. Oral Contraceptives and Ascorbic Acid. *American Journal of Clinical Nutrition* 28:5, 550–554, May 1975.

Rivers, J. M., and Devine, M. M. Plasma Ascorbic Acid Concentrations and Oral Contraceptives. *American Journal of Clinical Nutrition* 25:7, 684–689, July 1972.

Rolfe, E. J. Opening Remarks. In Birch, G. G., and Parker, K. J. *Vitamin C: Recent Aspects of Its Physiological and Technological Importance.* 1974. New York, Wiley.

Sahud, M. A., and Cohen, R. J. Effect of Aspirin Ingestion on Ascorbic-Acid Levels in Rheumatoid Arthritis. *Lancet* 1:7706, 937–938, 8 May 1971.

Science News. Editorial. March 29, 1980.

Smoking and Health: A Report of the Surgeon General. 1979. Rockville, Maryland, United States Department of Health, Education, and Welfare.

Spitzer, J. M., and Shapiro, S. The Effect of Salicylate Medication Upon the Urinary Excretion of Vitamin C. *American Journal of Digestive Diseases* 15:3, 80–84, March 1948.

United States Department of Health, Education, and Welfare. *Current Estimates: From the Health Interview Survey: United States 1978.* Series #10, #130, Vital and Health Statistics: Data from the National

Health Survey. DHEW Publication No. (PHS) 80-1551. November 1979. Hyattsville, Maryland, National Center for Health Statistics.

United States Department of Health, Education, and Welfare. *Use Habits Among Adults of Cigarettes, Coffee, Aspirin, and Sleeping Pills.* United States, 1976. Series 10, No. 131. DHEW Publication No. (PHS) 80-1559, October 1979. Hyattsville, Maryland, Office of Health Research, Statistics, and Technology, National Center for Health Statistics.

White, J. R., and Froeb, H. F. Small-Airways Dysfunction in Nonsmokers Chronically Exposed to Tobacco Smoke. *New England Journal of Medicine* 302:13, 720–723, March 27, 1980.

Wright, R. A. Nutritional Assessment. *Journal of the American Medical Association* 244:6, 559–560, 8 August 1980.

Wynn, V. Vitamins and Oral Contraceptive Use. *Lancet* 1:7906, 561–564, 8 March 1975.

Young, E. A., Brennan, E. H., and Irving, G. L. More Perspectives on Fast Foods. *Medical Times* 107:7, 23–29, July 1979.

3. How Not to Be Bugged by Infections

Anderson R., and Dittrich, O. C. Effects of Ascorbate on Leucocytes: Part IV. Increased Neutrophil Function and Clinical Improvement After Oral Ascorbate in Two Patients with Chronic Granulomatous Disease. *South African Medical Journal* 56:12, 476–480, 1 September 1979.

Anderson, R., Hay, I., Van Wyk, H., Oosthuizen, R., and Theron, A. The Effect of Ascorbate on Cellular Humoral Immunity in Asthmatic Children. *South African Medical Journal* 58:24, 974–977, 13 December 1980.

Anderson, R., Oosthuizen, R., Maritz, R., Theron, A., and Van Rensburg, A. J. The Effects of Increasing Weekly Doses of Ascorbate on Certain Cellular and Humoral Immune Functions in Normal Volunteers. *American Journal of Clinical Nutrition* 33:1, 71–76, January 1980.

Anderson, R., and Theron, A. Effects of Ascorbate on Leucocytes: Part III. In Vitro and In Vivo Stimulation of Abnormal Neutrophil Motility by Ascorbate. *South African Medical Journal* 56:11, 429–433, 8 September 1979.

Banic, S. Prevention of Rabies by Vitamin C. *Nature* 258:5531, 153–154, 13 November 1975.

Bouhuys, A. Colds and Antihistaminic Effects of Vitamin C. *New Eng-*

land Journal of Medicine 290:1, 633, 14 March 1974.

Boxer, L. A., Vanderbilt, B., Bonsib, S., Jersild, R., Yang, H. H., and Baehner, R. L. Enhancement of Chemotactic Response and Microtubule Assembly in Human Leukocytes by Ascorbic Acid. *Journal of Cellular Physiology* 100:1, 119–126, July 1979.

Cathcart, R. F., III. The Method of Determining Proper Doses of Vitamin C for the Treatment of Disease by Titrating to Bowel Tolerance. *Journal of Orthomolecular Psychiatry* 10:2, 125–132, March-April 1981.

Cell Organelle Defects Again Associated with Genetic Disease. *Journal of the American Medical Association* 238:6, 461–462, 8 August 1977.

Cheraskin, E., Ringsdorf, W. M., Jr., Michael, D. W., and Hicks, B. S. Daily Vitamin C Consumption and Reported Respiratory Findings. *International Journal for Vitamin and Nutrition Research* 43:1, 42–55, 1973.

Dahl, H., and Degre, M. The Effect of Ascorbic Acid on Production of Human Interferon and the Antiviral Activity In Vitro. *Acta Pathologica et Microbiologica Scandinavica* 84:5, 280–284, October 1976.

Foster, C. S., and Goetzl, E. J. Ascorbate Therapy in Impaired Neutrophil and Monocyte Chemotaxis with Atopy, Hyperimmunoglobulinemia E and Recurrent Infection. *Archives of Ophthalmology* 96:11, 2069–2072, November 1978.

Friedenberg, W. R., Marx, J. J., Jr., Hansen, R. L., and Haselby, R. C. Hyperimmunoglobulin E Syndrome: Response to Transfer Factor and Ascorbic Acid Therapy. *Clinical Immunology and Immunopathology* 12:2, 132–142, February 1979.

Goetzl, E. J., Wasserman, S. I., Gigli, I., and Austen, K. F. Enhancement of Random Migration and Chemotactic Response of Human Leukocytes by Ascorbic Acid. *Journal of Clinical Investigation* 53:3, 813–818, March 1974.

Holder, J. M. Vitamin C and Antibacterial Activity in Abnormal Tears. *Journal of Clinical Chiropractic* 2:2, 4–9, February 1978.

Horrobin, D. F., Oka, M., and Manku, M. S. The Regulation of Prostaglandin E_1 Formation: A Candidate for One of the Fundamental Mechanisms Involved in the Actions of Vitamin C. *Medical Hypotheses* 5:8, 849–858, August 1979.

International Comments. Vitamin C for Patients with Leprosy. *Journal of the American Medical Association* 233:2, 188, 14 July 1975.

Jackson, J. A. Ascorbic Acid Versus Allergies. *New York Journal of Dentistry* 42:7, 216–218, August–September 1972.

Kirkman, D. Vitamin C Protects Mothers, Unborn Babies, Doctor Says.

Scripps-Howard News Service, *Birmingham Post-Herald*, 8 July 1980.

Klenner, F. R. Observations on the Dose and Administration of Ascorbic Acid When Employed Beyond the Range of a Vitamin in Human Pathology. *Journal of Applied Nutrition* 23:3 and 4, 61–88, Winter 1971.

Kordansky, D. W., Rosenthal, R. R., and Norman, P. S. The Effect of Vitamin C on Antigen-Induced Bronchospasm. *Journal of Allergy and Clinical Immunology* 63:1, 61–64, January 1979.

Kreisman, H., Mitchell, C., and Bouhuys, A. Inhibition of Histamine-Induced Airway Constriction: Negative Results with Oxtriphylline and Ascorbic Acid. *Lung* 154:3, 223–229, 1977.

Leibovitz, B., and Siegel, B. Ascorbic Acid, Neutrophil Function, and the Immune Response. *International Journal for Vitamin and Nutrition Research* 48:2, 159–164, 1978.

Luberoff, B. J. Symptomectomy. A Chat with Robert Cathcart, M.D. *Chemtech* 8:2, 76–86, February 1978.

Manzella, J. P., and Roberts, N. J., Jr. Human Macrophage and Lymphocyte Responses to Mitogen Stimulation After Exposure to Influenza Virus, Ascorbic Acid and Hyperthermia. *Journal of Immunology* 123:5, 1940–1944, November 1979.

Matsuo, E., Skinsnes, O. K., and Chang, P. H. C. Acid Mucopholysaccharide Metabolism in Leprosy. 3. Hyaluronic Acid Mycobacterial Growth Enhancement, and Growth Suppression by Saccharic Acid and Vitamin C as Inhibitors of Beta-Glucuronidase. *International Journal of Leprosy* 43:1, 1–13, January–March 1975.

McCormick, W. J. Ascorbic Acid as a Chemotherapeutic Agent. *Archives of Pediatrics* 69:4, 151–155, April 1952.

Murata, A. Virucidal Activity of Vitamin C: Vitamin C for Prevention and Treatment of Viral Diseases. In Hasegawa, T., editor. *Proceedings of the First Intersectional Congress of the International Association of Microbiological Societies*, 1975, Volume III. Tokyo University Press. Pp. 432–442.

Nandi, B. K., Subramanian, N., Majumder, A. K., and Chatterjee, I. B. Effect of Ascorbic Acid on Detoxification of Histamine Under Stress Conditions. *Biochemical Pharmacology* 23:3, 643–647, 1 February 1974.

Nickey, K. E. Urinary pH: Effect of Prescribed Regimes of Cranberry Juice and Ascorbic Acid. *Archives of Physical Medicine and Rehabilitation* 56:12, 556, December 1975.

Panush, and Delafuenta, J. C. Cited by Yonemoto, R. H. Vitamin C and Immune Response. Presented at a symposium entitled "Vitamin C—

Its Pharmacologic Activity and Nutritional Aspects," March 1980, Mexico City, National Commission of Fruiticulture.

Pauling, L. The Case for Vitamin C in Maintaining Health and Preventing Disease. *Modern Medicine* 44:13, 68–72, 1 July 1976.

———. *Vitamin C, the Common Cold and the Flu.* 1976. San Francisco, W. H. Freeman.

Prinz, W., Bortz, R., Bregin, B., and Hersch, M. The Effect of Ascorbic Acid Supplementation on Some Parameters of the Human Immunological Defense System. *International Journal for Vitamin and Nutrition Research* 47:3, 248–257, 1977.

Rawal, B. D., McKay, G., and Blackhall, M. I. Inhibition of Pseudomonas Aeruginosa by Ascorbic Acid Acting Singly and in Combination with Antimicrobials: In-Vitro and In-Vivo Studies. *Medical Journal of Australia* 1:6, 169–174, 9 February 1974.

Rebora, A., Callegri, F., and Patrone, F. Neutrophil Dysfunction and Repeated Infections: Influence of Levamisole and Ascorbic Acid. *British Journal of Dermatology* 102:1, 49–56, January 1980.

Ries, P. W. *Acute Conditions, Incidence and Associated Disability, United States, July 1977–June 1978.* Vital and Health Statistics. Data from The National Health Survey; Series 10, 132, DHEW Publication No. (PHS) 79-1560.

Ringsdorf, W. M., Jr., and Cheraskin, E. Vitamin C and Antibiotics. *Journal of Oral Medicine* 35:1, 14–17, January–March 1980.

Rous, S. N. Symptomatic Treatment in Selected Cases of Urethritis. *New York State Journal of Medicine* 71:24, 2865–2866, 15 December 1971.

Schlesinger, A., and Schachter, E. N. The Attenuation of Exercise-Induced Bronchospasm by Ascorbic Acid. *Chest* 78:3, 538, September 1980.

Schwerdt, P. R., and Schwerdt, C. E. Effect of Ascorbic Acid on Rhinovirus Replication in WI-38 Cells. *Proceedings of the Society for Experimental Biology and Medicine* 148:4, 1237–1243, April 1975.

Slotkin, G. E., and Fletcher, R. S. Ascorbic Acid in Pulmonary Complications Following Prostatic Surgery: A Preliminary Report. *Journal of Urology* 52:6, 566–569, December 1944.

Stone, I. *The Healing Factor: Vitamin C Against Disease.* 1972. New York, Grosset and Dunlap.

Subramanian, N. Histamine Degradative Potential of Ascorbic Acid: Considerations and Evaluations. *Agents and Actions* 8:5, 484–487, 1978.

———, Nandi, B. K., Majumder, A. K., and Chatterjee, I. B. Role of L-

Ascorbic Acid on Detoxification of Histamine. *Biochemical Pharmacology* 22:13, 1671–1673, 1 July 1973.

Terezhalmy, G. T., Bottomley, W. K., and Pelleu, G. B. The Use of Water-Soluble Bioflavonoid–Ascorbic Acid Complex in the Treatment of Recurrent Herpes Labialis. *Oral Surgery, Oral Medicine, and Oral Pathology* 45:1, 56–62, January 1978.

Thomas, W. R., and Holt, P. G. Vitamin C and Immunity: An Assessment of the Evidence. *Clinical and Experimental Immunology* 32:2, 370–379, May 1978.

Thurman, G. B. Suppression of Immunological Responsivity in Guinea Pigs by Ascorbic Acid Depletion. Presented at a symposium entitled "Vitamin C—Its Pharmacologic Activity and Nutritional Aspects," March 1980, Mexico City, National Commission of Fruiticulture.

Valic, F., and Zuskin, E. Pharmacological Prevention of Acute Ventilatory Capacity Reduction in Flax Dust Exposure. *British Journal of Industrial Medicine* 30:4, 381–384, October 1973.

Vallance, S. Relationship Between Ascorbic Acid and Serum Proteins of the Immune System. *British Medicine Journal* 2:6084, 437–438, 13 August 1977.

Vitamin C Ups Resistance to Infection in Genetic Disease. *Medical News* 2:6, 13, 6 March 1978.

Wilson, C. W. M., Loh, H. S., and Watters, K. Vitamin C Metabolism and Atopic Allergy. *Clinical Allergy* 5:3, 317–324, September 1975.

Yonemoto, R. H. Vitamin C and Immune Response. Presented at a Symposium entitled "Vitamin C—Its Pharmacologic Activity and Nutritional Aspects," March 1980, Mexico City, National Commission of Fruiticulture.

Zuskin, E., Lewis, A. J., and Bouhuys, A. Inhibition of Histamine-Induced Airway Constriction by Ascorbic Acid. *Journal of Allergy and Clinical Immunology* 51:4, 218–226, April 1973.

Zuskin, E., Valic, F., and Bouhuys, A. Byssinosis and Airway Responses Due to Exposure to Textile Dust. *Lung* 154:1, 17–24, 1976.

4. Vitamin C: the Natural Healer

Afifi, A. M., Ellis, L., Huntsman, R. G., and Said, M. I. High Dose Ascorbic Acid in the Management of Thalassaemia Leg Ulcers—A Pilot Study. *British Journal of Dermatology* 92:3, 339–341, March 1975.

Bartlett, M., Jones, C. M., and Ryan, A. E. Vitamin C and Wound Healing. II. Ascorbic Acid Content and Tensile Strength of Healing

Wounds in Human Beings. *New England Journal of Medicine* 226:12, 474–481, March 1942.

Bourne, G. H. The Effect of Vitamin C on the Healing of Wounds. *Proceedings of the Nutrition Society* 4:3–4, 204–216, 1946.

Burr, R. G., and Rajan, K. T. Leucocyte Ascorbic Acid and Pressure Sores in Paraplegia. *British Journal of Nutrition* 28:2, 275–281, September 1972.

Cannon, W. B. *The Wisdom of the Body.* 1932. New York, W. W. Norton.

Cheraskin, E. The Ecology of Periodontal Disease. *Report Proceedings. Workshop on Diet, Nutrition and Periodontal Disease, American Society of Preventive Dentistry,* Sun Valley, Idaho, 7–27, 4–7 August 1974.

Collins, C. K., Lewis, A. E., Ringsdorf, W. M., Jr., and Cheraskin, E. Effect of Ascorbic Acid on Oral Healing in Guinea Pigs. *International Journal of Vitamin Research* 37:4, 492–495, 1967.

Elsas, L. J., Miller, R. L., and Pinnell, S. R. Inherited Human Collagen Lysyl Hydroxylase Deficiency: Ascorbic Acid Response. *Journal of Pediatrics* 92:3, 378–384, March 1978.

Gentile, A. *Physician Visits, Volume and Interval Since Last Visit, United States, 1975.* Vital and Health Statistics. Series 10, Data from the National Health Survey:128, DHEW publication (PHS)79-1556.

Givens, J. D. *Current Estimates from the Health Interview Survey, United States, 1978.* Vital and Health Statistics. Series 10, Data from the National Health Survey: 130, DHEW publication (PHS)80-1551.

Haupt, B. J. *Utilization of Short-Stay Hospitals, United States, 1978.* Vital and Health Statistics. Series 13, Data from the National Health Survey: 46, DHEW publication (PHS)80-1797.

Holmes, H. N. Shock. *Science* 96:2495, 384–386, 23 October 1942.

———. The Use of Vitamin C in Traumatic Shock. *Ohio State Medical Journal* 42:12, 1261–1264, December 1946.

Hunt, A. H. The Role of Vitamin C in Wound Healing. *British Journal of Surgery* 28:111, 436–461, January 1941.

Hunter, T., and Rajan, K. T. The Role of Ascorbic Acid in the Pathogenesis and Treatment of Pressure Sores. *Paraplegia* 8:4, 211–216, February 1971.

Irvin, T. T., Chattopadhyay, D. K., and Smythe, A. Ascorbic Acid Requirements in Postoperative Patients. *Surgery, Gynecology and Obstetrics* 147:1, 49–55, July 1978.

Khosla, V. M., and Gough, J. E. Evaluation of Three Techniques for the Management of Postextraction Third Molar Sockets. *Oral Surgery* 31:2, 189–198, February 1971.

Levinson, R. A., Paterson, C. A., and Pfister, R. R. Ascorbic Acid Prevents Corneal Ulceration and Perforation Following Experimental Alkali Burns. *Investigative Ophthalmology and Visual Science* 15:12, 986–993, December 1976.

Passmore, R. How Vitamin C Deficiency Injures the Body. *Nutrition Today* 12:2, 6–11, 27–31, March-April 1977.

Pfister, R. R., and Paterson, C. A. Additional Clinical and Morphological Observations on the Favorable Effect of Ascorbate in Experimental Ocular Alkali Burns. *Investigative Ophthalmology and Visual Science* 16:6, 478–487, June 1977.

Pfister, R. R., Paterson, C. A., and Hayes, S. A. Topical Ascorbate Decreases the Incidence of Corneal Ulceration After Experimental Alkali Burns. *Investigative Ophthalmology and Visual Science* 17:10, 1019–1024, October 1978.

Ringsdorf, W. M., Jr., and Cheraskin, E. Vitamin C and Human Wound Healing. *Oral Surgery, Oral Medicine, Oral Pathology* 53:3, 231–236, March 1982.

Schwartz, P. L. Ascorbic Acid in Wound Healing—A Review. *Journal of the American Dietetic Association* 56:6, 497–503, June 1970.

Shukla, S. P. Plasma and Urinary Ascorbic Acid Levels in the Postoperative Period. *Experienta* 25:7, 704, 1969.

Silvetti, A. N., Krejei-Simmons, C., and Schwartz, D. Accelerated Wound Healing and Infection Control Through the Topical Application of Nutrients. *Federation Proceedings* 40:3, Part II, 922 (abstract #3929), 1 March 1981.

Taylor, T. V., Rimmer, S., Day, B., Butcher, J., and Dymock, I. W. Ascorbic Acid Supplementation in the Treatment of Pressure-Sores. *Lancet* 2:7880, 544–546, 7 September 1974.

Vitamin C May Enhance Healing of Caustic Corneal Burns. *Journal of the American Medical Association* 243:7, 623, 15 February 1980.

Wolfer, J. A., Farmer, C. J., Carroll, W. W., and Manshardt, D. O. An Experimental Study in Wound Healing in Vitamin C Depleted Human Subjects. *Surgery, Gynecology and Obstetrics* 84:1, 1–15, January 1947.

5. The Thermostat in *Your* Energy Crisis

Hindson, T. C. Ascorbic Acid for Prickly Heat. *Lancet* 1:7556, 1347–1348, 22 June 1968.

Hindson, T. C., and Worsley, D. E. The Effects of Administration of Ascorbic Acid in Experimentally Induced Miliaria and Hypohidrosis in Volunteers. *British Journal of Dermatology* 81:3, 226–227, March 1969.

Krasnopevtsev, V. M., Levin, A. I., Jushko, Y. K., Shevyreva, N. A., Khristenko, P. P., Maksimenko, R. G., and Djachenko, I. F. The Role of Nutrition in Adaptation of the Population to the Conditions of the Extreme North. (abstract) *Nutrition Today* 15:1, 30, January–February 1980.

Livingstone, S. D. Changes in Cold-Induced Vasodilation During Arctic Exercises. *Journal of Applied Physiology* 40:3, 455–457, March 1976.

——. Effect of Vitamin C on Cold-Induced Vasodilatation. *Lancet* 2:7980, 319–320, 7 August 1976.

Nakamura, M., Kawagoe, T., Ogino, Y., Nishiyama, K., Ichikawa, H., and Sugahara, K. Experimental Study on the Effect of Vitamin C on the Basal Metabolism and Resistance to Cold in Human Beings. *Tohoky Journal of Experimental Medicine* 92:2, 207–219, June 1967.

Pawley, R. E., and Berry, C. A. Cited by Stern, R. I. Relief of Prickly Heat with Vitamin C. *Journal of the American Medical Association* 145:3, 175, 20 January 1951.

Poda, G. A. Vitamin C for Heat Symptoms? *Annals of Internal Medicine* 91:4, 657, October 1979.

Ringsdorf, W. M., Jr., and Cheraskin, E. Vitamin C and Tolerance of Heat and Cold: Human Evidence. *Journal of Orthomolecular Psychiatry* 11:2, 128–131, Second Quarter 1982.

Stern, R. I. Relief of Prickly Heat with Vitamin C. *Journal of the American Medical Association* 145:3, 175, 20 January 1951.

Strydom, N. B., Kotze, H. F., VanDerWalt, W. H., and Rogers, G. G. Effect of Ascorbic Acid on Rate of Heat Acclimatization. *Journal of Applied Physiology* 41:2, 202–205, August 1976.

Weaver, W. L. The Prevention of Heat Prostration by Use of Vitamin C. *Southern Medical Journal* 41:5, 479–481, May 1948.

6. Pain and Vitamin C

Basu, T. K., Smethurst, M., Gillett, M. B., Donaldson, D., Jordan, S. J., Williams, D. C., and Hicklin, J. A. Ascorbic Acid Therapy for the Relief of Bone Pain in Paget's Disease. *Acta Vitaminologica et Enzymologica* 32:1–4, 45–49, 1978.

Bonham, G. S. *Use Habits of Cigarettes, Coffee, Aspirin, and Sleeping Pills, United States 1976.* Vital and Health Statistics: Series 10, Data from the National Health Survey; 131, DHEW publication number (PHS) 80-1559.

Cameron, E., and Baird, G. M. Ascorbic Acid and Dependence on Opiates in Patients with Advanced and Disseminated Cancer. *Journal of International Research Communications* 1:6, 38, August 1973.

Cameron, E., and Campbell, A. The Orthomolecular Treatment of Cancer. II. Clinical Trial of High-Dose Ascorbic Acid in Advanced Human Cancer. *Chemical-Biological Interactions* 9:4, 285–315, October 1974.

Gentile, A. Physician Visits, Volume and Interval Since Last Visit, United States, 1975. Vital and Health Statistics: Series 10, Data from the National Health Survey; 128, DHEW publication number (PHS) 79-1556.

Greenwood, J., Jr. Optimum Vitamin C Intake as a Factor in the Preservation of Disc Integrity. *Medical Annals of the District of Columbia* 33:6, 274–276, June 1964.

Gupte, S. R., and Savant, N. S. Post Suxamethonium Pain and Vitamin C. *Anaesthesia* 26:4, 436–440, October 1971.

Haupt, B. J. *Utilization of Short-Stay Hospitals, United States, 1978.* Vital and Health Statistics: Series 13, Data from the National Health Survey; 46, DHEW publication number (PHS) 80-1797.

Jack, S. S. *Current Estimates from the National Health Interview Survey: United States, 1980.* Vital and Health Statistics: Series 10, Data from the National Health Survey; 139, DHHS publication number (PHS) 82-1567.

Kurz, D., and Eyring, E. J. Effects of Vitamin C on Osteogenesis Imperfecta. *Pediatrics* 54:1, 56–61, July 1974.

Syed, I. H. Muscle Stiffness and Vitamin C. *British Medical Journal* 2:5508, 304, 30 July 1966.

Winterfeldt, E. A., Eyring, E. J., and Vivian, V. M. Ascorbic Acid Treatment for Osteogenesis Imperfecta. *Lancet* 1:7660, 1347–1348, 20 June 1970.

7. Colds: from Chaos to Conviction

Anderson, T. W. Vitamin C and the Common Cold. *Journal of the Medical Society of New Jersey* 76:11, 765–766, October 1979.

——. Vitamin C: Report of Trials with Massive Doses. In White, P. L., and Selvey, N., editors, *Proceedings Western Hemisphere Nutrition Congress IV.* Bal Harbour, Florida, 19–22 August 1974. Acton, Massachusetts, Publishing Sciences Group, Inc. Pp. 92–96.

Baird, I. M., Hughes, R. E., Wilson, H. K., Davies, J. E. W., and Howard, A. N. The Effects of Ascorbic Acid and Flavonoids on the Occurrence of Symptoms Normally Associated with the Common Cold. *American Journal of Clinical Nutrition* 32:8, 1686–1690, August 1979.

Bouhuys, A. Colds and Antihistaminic Effects of Vitamin C. *New England Journal of Medicine* 290:1, 633, 14 March 1974.

Cathcart, R. F., III. The Method of Determining Proper Doses of Vitamin C for the Treatment of Disease by Titrating to Bowel Tolerance. *Journal of Orthomolecular Psychiatry* 10:2, 125–132, March-April 1981.

Cheraskin, E., Ringsdorf, W. M., Jr., Michael, D. W., and Hicks, B. S. Daily Vitamin C Consumption and Reported Respiratory Findings. *International Journal for Vitamin and Nutrition Research* 43:1, 42–55, 1973.

Coulehan, J. L. Ascorbic Acid and the Common Cold. *Postgraduate Medicine* 66:3, 153–155, 157–158, 160, September 1979.

Editorial. Cold Concern. *Executive Fitness Newsletter* 6:21, 11 October 1975.

Klenner, F. R. Observations on the Dose and Administration of Ascorbic Acid When Employed Beyond the Range of a Vitamin in Human Pathology. *Journal of Applied Nutrition* 23:3–4, 61–88, Winter 1971.

Lewin, S. *Vitamin C: Its Molecular Biology and Medical Potential.* 1976. New York, Academic Press.

Marckwell, N. W. Vitamin C in the Prevention of Colds. *Medical Journal of Australia* 2:26, 777–778, 27 December 1947.

McCormick, W. J. Ascorbic Acid as a Chemotherapeutic Agent. *Archives of Pediatrics* 69:4, 151–155, April 1952.

Pauling, L. The Case for Vitamin C in Maintaining Health and Preventing Disease. *Modern Medicine* 44:13, 68–72, 1 July 1976.

——. *Vitamin C, the Common Cold and the Flu.* 1976. San Francisco, W. H. Freeman.

Regnier, E. The Administration of Large Doses of Ascorbic Acid in the Prevention and Treatment of the Common Cold. Part I. *Review of Allergy* 22:9, 835–846, September 1968. Part II. *Review of Allergy* 22:10, 948–956, October 1968.

Ries, P. W. *Acute Conditions, Incidence and Associated Disability, United States, July 1977—June 1978.* Vital and Health Statistics. Data from the National Health Survey; Series 10,132, DHEW publication number (PHS)79-1560.

Ruskin, S. L. Calcium Cevitamate (Calcium Ascorbate) in the Treatment of Acute Rhinitis. *Annals of Otology, Rhinology and Laryngology.* 47:2, 502–511, June 1938.

Schwerdt, P. R., and Schwerdt, C. E. Effect of Ascorbic Acid on Rhinovirus Replication in WI-38 Cells. *Proceedings of the Society for Experimental Biology and Medicine* 148:4, 1237–1243, April 1975.

Stone, I. *The Healing Factor: Vitamin C Against Disease.* 1972. New York, Grosset and Dunlap.

8. Pumping C

Allport, S. Long Term Toxic Effects from Clofibrate Reported. *Medical News* 4:20, 2, 8 December 1980.

Armstrong, B. K., Mann, J. I., Adelstein, A. M., and Eskin, F. Commodity Consumption and Ischemic Heart Disease Mortality with Special Reference to Dietary Practices. *Journal of Chronic Diseases* 28:9, 455–469, October 1975.

Bordia, A. The Effect of Vitamin C on Blood Lipids, Fibrinolytic Activity, and Platelet Adhesiveness in Patients with Coronary Artery Disease. *Atherosclerosis* 35:2, 181–187, February 1980.

——, Paliwal, D. K., Jain, K., and Kothari, L. K. Acute Effect of Ascorbic Acid on Fibrinolytic Activity. *Atherosclerosis* 30:4, 351–354, August 1978.

Boukhris, R., Khaznaji, M., Akef, N., and BeuAyed, H. Lipemia, Uricemia, and Vitamin C. *Tunisie Medicale* 51:1, 25–29, January–February 1973.

Bronte-Stewart, B., Roberts, B., and Wells, V. M. Serum Cholesterol in Vitamin C Deficiency in Man. *British Journal of Nutrition* 17:1, 61–68, 1963.

Cheraskin, E., and Ringsdorf, W. M., Jr. Another Look at the "Ideal" Serum Cholesterol Level? *Archives of Internal Medicine* 140:4, 580–581, April 1980.

——, ——, and Hicks, B. S. Daily Vitamin C Consumption and Reported Cardiovascular Findings. *Journal of the International Academy of Preventive Medicine* 1:1, 31–44, Spring 1974.

Clemetson, C. A. B. Some Thoughts on the Epidemiology of Cardiovascular Disease (With Special Reference to Women "On the Pill"), Role of Ascorbic Acid. *Medical Hypotheses* 5:8, 825–834, August 1979.

Davies, J. D. G., and Newsom, J. Ascorbic Acid and Cholesterol Levels in Pastoral Peoples in Kenya. *American Journal of Clinical Nutrition* 27:10, 1039–1042, October 1974.

Dunnigan, M. G., Harland, W. A., and Fyfe, T. Seasonal Incidence and Mortality of Ischaemic Heart Disease. *Lancet* 2:7677, 793–797, 17 October 1970.

Eastham, R. D., and Avis, P. R. D. Seasonal Fluctuation in Adhesive

Platelets During Long-Term Anticoagulant Therapy. *British Journal of Haematology* 12:1, 39–43, January 1966.

Follis, R. H., Jr. Effect of Mechanical Force on the Skeletal Lesions in Acute Scurvy in Guinea Pigs. *Archives of Pathology* 34:4, 579–582, April 1943.

——. Sudden Death in Infants with Scurvy. *Journal of Pediatrics* 20:3, 347–351, March 1942.

Fyfe, T., Dunnigan, M. G., Hamilton, E., and Rae, R. J. Seasonal Variation in Serum Lipids and Incidence and Mortality of Ischaemic Heart Disease. *Journal of Atherosclerosis Research* 8:3, 591–596, May–June 1968.

Gentile, A. *Physician Visits, Volume and Interval Since Last Visit, United States, 1975.* Vital and Health Statistics: Series 10, Data from the National Health Survey; 128, DHEW publication number (PHD) 79–1556.

Ginter, E. Cholesterol: Vitamin C Controls Its Transformation to Bile Acids. *Science* 179:74, 702–704, 16 February 1973.

——. Decline of Coronary Mortality in the United States and Vitamin C. *American Journal of Clinical Nutrition* 32:3, 511–512, March 1979.

——. Marginal Vitamin C Deficiency, Lipid Metabolism and Atherogenesis. *Advances in Lipid Research* 16, 167–220, 1978.

——. The Role of Vitamin C in Lipid Metabolism. Presented at a symposium entitled "Vitamin C—Its Pharmacologic Activity and Nutritional Aspects," March 1980, Mexico City, Mexico, National Commission of Fruiticulture.

——. Vitamin C, Blood Cholesterol, and Atherosclerosis. *American Laboratory* 8:6, 21–26, 28–29, June 1976.

——, Cerna, O., Budlovsky, J., Balaz, V., Hruba, F., Roch, V., and Sasko, E. Effect of Ascorbic Acid on Plasma Cholesterol in Humans in a Long-Term Experiment. *International Journal for Vitamin and Nutrition Research* 47:2, 123–134, 1977.

——, Kajaba, I., and Nizner, O. The Effect of Ascorbic Acid on Cholesterolemia in Healthy Subjects with Seasonal Deficit of Vitamin C. *Nutrition and Metabolism* 12: 76–86, 1970.

Hanck, A. B. Plasma Cholesterol Level in Healthy Subjects and Its Modification by Large Doses of L(+)−Ascorbic Acid. *Zeitschrift für Ernährungswissenschaft* 12:2, 152–158, June 1973.

Haupt, B. *Utilization of Short-Stay Hospitals, 1978.* Data from the National Health Survey: Series 13; 46, DHEW publication number (PHS) 80–1797.

Horsey, J., Livesley, B. and Dickerson, J. W. T. Ischaemic Heart Disease and Aged Patients. Effects of Ascorbic Acid on Lipoproteins. *Journal of Human Nutrition* 35:1, 53–58, February 1981.

Hume, R., Weyers, E., Rowan, T., Reid, D. S., and Hillis, W. S. Leukocyte Ascorbic Acid Levels After Acute Myocardial Infarction. *British Heart Journal* 34:3, 238–243, March 1972.

Knox, E. G. Ischaemic-Heart-Disease, Mortality and Dietary Intake of Calcium. *Lancet* 1:7818, 1465–1467, 30 June 1973.

Krebs, H. A. The Sheffield Experiment on the Vitamin C Requirement of Human Adults. *Proceedings of the Nutrition Society* 12:2, 237–246, 1953.

Krumdieck, C., and Butterworth, C. E., Jr. Ascorbate-Cholesterol-Lecithin Interactions: Factors of Potential Importance in the Pathogenesis of Atherosclerosis. *American Journal of Clinical Nutrition* 27:8, 866–876, August 1974.

Lopez-S., A. Vitamin C and Cardiovascular Disease. Presented at a symposium entitled "Vitamin C—Its Pharmacologic Activity and Nutritional Aspects," March 1980, Mexico City, Mexico, National Commission of Fruiticulture.

Magoon, C. E. U.S. Food Intake Has More Nutritional Value Than in 1965. *United Fresh Fruit and Vegetable Association Monthly Supply Letter*, January 1980.

Morrison, L. M., and Enrick, N. L. Coronary Heart Disease: Reduction of Death Rate by Chondroitin Sulfate A. *Angiology* 24:5, 269–287, May 1973.

Paul, O., Lepper, M. H., Phelan, W. H., Dupertius, G. W., MacMillan, A., McKean, H., and Park, H. A Longitudinal Study of Coronary Heart Disease. *Circulation* 28:1, 20–31, July 1963.

Pfister, R. R., and Paterson, C. A. Additional Clinical and Morphological Observations on the Favorable Effect of Ascorbate in Experimental Ocular Alkali Burns. *Investigative Ophthalmology and Visual Science* 16:6, 478–487, June 1977.

Ramirez, J., and Flowers, N. C. Leukocyte Ascorbic Acid and Its Relationship to Coronary Artery Disease in Man. *American Journal of Clinical Nutrition* 33:10, 2079–2087, October 1980.

Sarji, K. E., Kleinfelder, J., Brewington, P., Gonzalez, J., Hempling, H., and Colwell, J. A. Decreased Platelet Vitamin C in Diabetes Mellitus: Possible Role in Hyperaggregation. *Thrombosis Research* 15:5–6, 639–650, 1979.

Shafar, J. Rapid Reversion of Electrocardiographic Abnormalities After Treatment in Two Cases of Scurvy. *Lancet* 2:7508, 176–178, 22 July 1967.

Shimizu, M., Hatta, Y., Hayashi, H., Itokawa, M., Yanagisawa, Y., Otani, T., and Nakachi, N. Effect of Ascorbic Acid on Fibrinolysis. *Acta Haematologica Japonica* 33:1, 137–148, February 1970.

Simonson, E., and Keys, A. Research in Russia on Vitamins and Atherosclerosis. *Circulation* 24:5, 1239–1248, November 1961.

Sokoloff, B., Mori, M., Saelhof, C. C., Wrzolek, T., and Imai, T. Aging, Atherosclerosis and Ascorbic Acid Metabolism. *Journal of the American Geriatrics Society* 14:12, 1239–1260, December 1966.

Spittle, C. R. The Action of Vitamin C on Blood Vessels. *American Heart Journal* 88:3, 387–388, September 1974.

——. Atherosclerosis and Vitamin C. *Lancet* 2:7737, 1280–1281, 11 December 1971.

——. Atherosclerosis and Vitamin C. *Lancet* 1:7754, 798, 8 April 1972.

——. Vitamin C and Deep-Vein Thrombosis. *Lancet* 2:7822, 199–201, 28 July 1973.

——. Vitamin C and Myocardial Infarction. *Lancet* 2:679, 931, 31 October 1970.

Stamler, J. *Lipids and Coronary Heart Disease.* 1979. New York, Raven Press. P. 25.

Taylor, T. V., Raftery, A. T., Elder, J. B., Loveday, C., Dymock, I. W., Gibbs, A. C. C., Jeacock, J., Lucas, S. B., and Pell, M. A. Leucocyte Ascorbate Levels and Postoperative Deep Venous Thrombosis. *British Journal of Surgery* 66:8, 583–585, August 1979.

Thomas, C. B., Holljes, H. W. D., and Eisenberg, F. F. Observations on Seasonal Variations in Total Serum Cholesterol Level Among Healthy Young Prisoners. *Annals of Internal Medicine* 54:3, 413–430, March 1961.

Vallance, B. D., Hume, R., and Weyers, E. Reassessment of Changes in Leucocyte and Serum Ascorbic Acid After Acute Myocardial Infarction. *British Heart Journal* 40:1, 64–68, January 1978.

Veshima, H., Iida, M., and Komachi, Y. Is It Desirable to Reduce Total Serum Cholesterol Level as Low as Possible? *Preventive Medicine* 8:1, 104–105, January 1979.

Willis, G. C. An Experimental Study of the Intimal Ground Substance in Atherosclerosis. *Canadian Medical Association Journal* 69:1, 17–22, July 1953.

——. The Reversibility of Atherosclerosis. *Canadian Medical Association Journal* 77:2, 106–109, 15 July 1957.

Willis, G. C., and Fishman, S. Ascorbic Acid Content of Human Arterial Tissue. *Canadian Medical Association Journal* 72:7, 500–503, 1 April 1955.

Willis, G. C., Light, A. W., and Gow, W. S. Serial Arteriography in

Atherosclerosis. *Canadian Medical Association Journal* 71:6, December 1954.

9. Sugar Is Sweet—Except in Diabetes

Colwell, J. A., and Lizarralde, G. *Diabetes and Metabolic Disorders: Continuing Education Review.* 1975. Flushing, New York, Medical Examination Publishing Company.

Cox, B. D., Whichelow, M. J., Butterfield, W. J. H., and Nicholas, P. Peripheral Vitamin C Metabolism in Diabetics and Non-Diabetics: Effect of Intra-Arterial Insulin. *Clinical Science & Molecular Medicine* 47:1, 63–72, July 1974.

Dice, J. F., and Daniel, C. W. The Hypoglycemic Effect of Ascorbic Acid in a Juvenile-Onset Diabetic. *Journal of the International Research Communications* 1:1, 41, March 1973.

Fajans, S. S. What Is Diabetes? Definition, Diagnosis and Course. *Medical Clinics of North America* 55:4, 793–805, July 1971.

Ginter, E., Zdichynec, B., Holzerova, O., Ticha, E., Kobza, R., Koziakova, M., Cerna, O., Ozion, L., Hruba, F., Novakova, V., Sasko, E., and Gaher, M. Hypocholesterolemic Effect of Ascorbic Acid in Maturity-Onset Diabetes Mellitus. *International Journal for Vitamin and Nutrition Research* 48:4, 368–373, 1978.

Hjorth, P. The Influence of Vitamin C on Carbohydrate Metabolism. *Acta Medica Scandinavica* 105:1–2, 67–72, 1940.

Köbberling, J., and Greutzfeldt, W. Diabetes Mellitus: A New Look at Diagnostic Criteria. *Diabetologica* 17:4, 263–264, October 1979.

Krall, L. P. *Joslin Diabetes Manual.* Eleventh Edition. 1978. Philadelphia, Lea & Febiger.

Nuttall, F. Q., and Brunzell, J. D. Principles of Nutrition and Dietary Recommendations for Individuals with Diabetes Mellitus: 1979. Report of the American Diabetes Association. *Journal of the American Dietetic Association* 75:5, 527–530, November 1979.

Pfleger, R., and Scholl, F. Diabetes and Vitamin C. *Wien Archives of Internal Medicine* 31: 219–230, 1937. Cited by Dykes, H. M., and Meier, P. Ascorbic Acid and the Common Cold. Evaluation of Its Efficacy and Toxicity. *Journal of the American Medical Association* 231:10, 1073–1079, 10 March 1975.

Sayetta, R. B., and Murphy, R. S. Summary of Current Diabetes-Related Data from the National Center for Health Statistics. *Diabetes Care* 2:2, 105–119, March-April 1979.

Secher, K. The Bearing of the Ascorbic Acid Content of the Blood on the

Course of the Blood Sugar Curve. *Acta Medica Scandinavica* 110:2–3, 255–265, 1942.

Setyaadmadja, A. T. S. H., Cheraskin, E., and Ringsdorf, W. M., Jr. Ascorbic Acid and Carbohydrate Metabolism: I. The Cortisone Glucose Tolerance Test. *Journal of the American Geriatrics Society* 13:10, 924–934, October 1965.

———. Ascorbic Acid and Carbohydrate Metabolism: II. Effect of Supervised Sucrose Drinks Upon Two-Hour Postprandial Blood Glucose in Terms of Vitamin C State. *Journal Lancet* 87:1, 18–21, January 1967.

Sigal, A., and King, C. G. The Influence of Vitamin C Deficiency Upon the Resistance of Guinea Pigs to Diphtheria Toxin: Glucose Tolerance. *Journal of Pharmacology and Experimental Therapeutics* 61:1, 1–9, September 1937.

———. The Relationship of Vitamin C to Glucose Tolerance in the Guinea Pig. *Journal of Biological Chemistry* 116:2, 489-492, December 1936.

Sylvest, O. The Effect of Ascorbic Acid on the Carbohydrate Metabolism. *Acta Medica Scandinavica* 110:2–3, 183–196, 1942.

West, K. M. Substantial Differences in the Diagnostic Criteria Used by Diabetes Experts. *Diabetes* 24:7, 641–644, July 1975.

10. The Two C's in Cancer

American Cancer Society. *Cancer Facts and Figures, 1980*. 777 Third Avenue, New York, N.Y. 10017.

Archer, M. C., Tannenbaum, S. R., Tan, T.-Y., and Weisman, M. Reaction of Nitrite with Ascorbate and Its Relation to Nitrosamine Formation. *Journal of the National Cancer Institute* 54:4, 1203–1205, May 1975.

Bodansky, O., Wroblewski, F., and Markardt, B. Concentrations of Ascorbic Acid in Plasma and White Cells of Patients with Cancer and Non-Cancerous Chronic Disease. *Cancer Research* 11:4, 238, April 1951.

Bram, S., Froussard, P., Guichard, M., Jasmin, C., Augery, Y., Sinoussi-Barre, F., and Wray, W. Vitamin C. Preferential Toxicity for Malignant Melanoma Cells. *Nature* 284:5757, 629–631, 17 April 1980.

Briggs, M. H. Vitamin C in the Buffy Coat in Leukemia. *Medical Journal Australia* 1:5, 152, 2 February 1974.

Cameron, E., and Campbell, A. The Orthomolecular Treatment of Cancer. II. Clinical Trial of High-Dose Ascorbic Acid Supplements in Advanced Human Cancer. *Chemical-Biological Interactions* 9:4, 285–315, October 1974.

Cameron, E., and Jack, T. The Orthomolecular Treatment of Cancer. III. Reticulum Cell Sarcoma: Double Complete Regression Induced by High Dose Ascorbic Acid Therapy. *Chemical-Biological Interactions* 11:5, 387–393, November 1975.

Cameron, E., and Pauling, L. Ascorbic Acid and the Glycosaminoglycans: An Orthomolecular Approach to Cancer and Other Diseases. *Oncology* 27:2, 181–192, 1973.

———. The Orthomolecular Treatment of Cancer. I. The Role of Ascorbic Acid in Host Resistance. *Chemical-Biological Interactions* 9:4, 273–283, October 1974.

———. Supplemental Ascorbate in the Supportive Treatment of Cancer: Prolongation of Survival Times in Terminal Human Cancer. *Proceedings of the National Academy of Sciences* 73:10, 3685–3689, October 1976.

———. Supplemental Ascorbate in the Supportive Treatment of Cancer: Reevaluation of Prolongation of Survival Times in Terminal Human Cancer. *Proceedings of the National Academy of Sciences* 75:9, 4538–4542, September 1978.

Cameron, E., and Leibovitz, B. Ascorbic Acid and Cancer: A Review. *Cancer Research* 39:3, 663–681, March 1979.

Cameron, E., and Rotman, D. Ascorbic Acid, Cell Proliferation, and Cancer. *Lancet* 1:749, 542, 4 March 1972.

Clayson, D. E. Nutrition and Experimental Carcinogenesis: A Review. Paper presented at the Conference on Nutrition in the Causation of Cancer. Key Biscayne, Fla., May 1975.

Creagan, E. T., Moertel, C. G., O'Fallon, J. R., Schutt, A. J., O'Connell, M. J., Rubin, J., and Frytak, S. Failure of High-Dose Vitamin C (Ascorbic Acid) Therapy to Benefit Patients with Advanced Cancer: A Controlled Trial. *New England Journal of Medicine* 301:13, 687–690, 27 September 1979.

DeCosse, J. J., Adams, M. B., Kuzma, J. F., LoGerfo, P., and Condon, R. E. Effect of Ascorbic Acid on Rectal Polyps in Patients with Familial Polyposis. *Surgery* 78:5, 608–612, November 1975.

Doeschuk, B. Sodium Nitrite: Exploring Alternatives. *Nutrition Action*, January 1976.

Editorial. Ascorbic Acid: An Anticancer Vitamin. *Medical World News* 9:25, 24, 21 June 1968.

Editorial. Do Vitamins C and E Prevent Cancer of Large Bowel? *Medical World News* 19:15, 24, 24 July 1978.

Editorial. Nitrites, Drugs and Drinking Water. *Science News* 108, 13 September 1975.

Endo, H., Ishizawa, M., Endo, T., Takahashi, K., Utsunomiya, T., Kinoshita, H., Hidaka, K., and Baba, T. A Possible Process of Conversion of Food Components to Gastric Carcinogens. In Hiatt, H. H., Watson, J. D., and Watson, J. A., Editors. *Origins of Human Cancer*. 1977. New York, Cold Spring Harbor Laboratory. Pp. 1591–1607.

Farber, E. Vitamin C and Cancer Research. Presented at a symposium entitled "Vitamin C—Its Pharmacologic Activity and Nutritional Aspects," March 1980, Mexico City, Mexico, National Commission of Fruiticulture.

Farrah, G. A. Supplemental Ascorbate Cancer Types Related to Number of Survival Days (Rank Order). *The Linus Pauling Institute of Science and Medicine Newsletter* 1:10, 3, Winter 1980.

Friedman, R. M., and Pastan, I. Interferon and Cyclic 3^1, 5^1-Adenosine Monophosphate: Potentiation of Antiviral Activity. *Biochemical and Biophysical Research Communications* 36:5, 735–740, 22 August 1969.

Goth, A., and Littman, I. Ascorbic Acid Content in Human Cancer Tissue. *Cancer Research* 8:8, 349–351, August 1948.

Greer, E. Alcoholic Cirrhosis Complicated by Polycythemia Vera and Then Myelogenous Leukemia and Tolerance of Large Doses of Vitamin C. *Medical Times* 82:11, 865–868, November 1954.

Griffiths, J. D., McKinna, J. A., Rowbotham, H. D., Tsolakidis, P., and Salsbury, A. J. Carcinoma of the Colon and Rectum; Circulating Malignant Cells and Five Year Survival. *Cancer* 31:1, 226–236, January 1973.

Hill, M. J. The Etiology of Colon Cancer. *CRC Critical Reviews in Toxicology* 4:1, 31–82, October 1975.

Kakar, S., and Wilson, C. W. M. Ascorbic Acid Metabolism in Human Cancer. *Proceedings of the Nutrition Society* 33:3, 110A, December 1974.

Kamm, J. J., Dashman, T., Conney, A. H., and Burns, J. J. Effect of Ascorbic Acid on Amine-Nitrite Toxicity. *Annals of the New York Academy of Sciences* (Second Conference on Vitamin C) 258, 169–174, 1975.

Klein, S. The Role of Vitamin C in the Prevention and Therapy of Cancer. *Journal of the International Academy of Preventive Medicine* 5:2, 9–28, 1978.

Koch, C. J., Howell, R. L., and Biaglow, J. E. Ascorbate Anion Potentiates Cytotoxicity of Nitro-Aromatic Compounds Under Hypoxic and Anoxic Conditions. *British Journal of Cancer* 39:2, 321–329, March 1979.

Krasner, N., and Dymock, I. W. Ascorbic Acid Deficiency in Malignant

Diseases: A Clinical and Biochemical Study. *British Journal of Cancer* 30:2, 142–145, August 1974.

Lakritz, L., Simenhoff, M. L., Dunn, S. R., and Fiddler, W. N-Nitrosodimethyamine in Human Blood. *Food and Cosmetics Toxicology* 18:1, 77–79, February 1980.

Lewin, S. *Vitamin C: Its Molecular Biology and Medical Potential.* 1979. New York, Academic Press. Pp. 160–165.

Lijinsky, W., and Epstein, S. S. Nitrosamines as Environmental Carcinogens. *Nature* 25:5227, 21–23, 3 January 1970.

Marquardt, H., Rufino, R., and Weisburger, J. H. Mutagenic Activity of Nitrite-Treated Foods: Human Stomach Cancer May Be Related to Dietary Factors. *Science* 196:4293, 1000–1001, 27 May 1977.

——. On the Etiology of Gastric Cancer: Mutagenicity of Food Extracts After Incubation with Nitrite. *Food and Cosmetics Toxicology* 15:2, 97–100, April 1977.

Medical News. Nitrosamines Look More Like Human Cancer Villains. *Journal of the American Medical Association* 238:1, 15–21, 4 July 1977.

Mirvish, S. S. Blocking the Formation of N-Nitroso Compounds with Ascorbic Acid in Vitro and in Vivo. *Annals of the New York Academy of Sciences* (Second Conference on Vitamin C) 258, 175–180, 1975.

——, Wallcave, L., Eagen, M., and Shubik, P. Ascorbic-Nitrite Reaction: Possible Means of Blocking the Formation of Carcinogenic N-Nitroso Compounds. *Science* 177:4043, 65–68, 7 July 1972.

Morishige, F., and Murata, A. Prolongation of Survival Times in Terminal Human Cancer by Administration of Supplemental Ascorbate. *Journal of the International Academy of Preventive Medicine* 5:1, 47–52, 1978.

Park, C. H., Amare, M., Savin, M. A., and Hogstraten, B. Growth Suppression of Human Leukemic Cells in Vitro by L-Ascorbic Acid. *Cancer Research* 40:4, 1062–1065, April 1980.

Pauling, L. *Vitamin C and Cancer.* 1979. New York, W. W. Norton.

Poydock, M. E., Tardon, J. C., Gallina, D., Ferro, V., and Heher, C. Inhibiting Effect of Vitamins C and B_{12} on the Mitotic Activity of Ascites Tumors. *Experimental Cell Biology.* 47:3, 210–217, 1979.

Prasad, K. N., Sinha, P. K., Ramanujam, M., and Sakamoto, A. Sodium Ascorbate Potentiates the Growth Inhibiting Effect of Certain Agents on Neuroblastoma Cells in Culture. *Proceedings of the National Academy of Sciences* 76:2, 829–832, February 1979.

Raineri, R., and Weisburger, H. J. Reduction of Gastric Carcinogens with Ascorbic Acid. *Annals of the New York Academy of Sciences* (Second Conference on Vitamin C) 258, 181–189, 1975.

Ryan, W. L., and Heidrick, M. L. Inhibition of Cell Growth in Vitro by Adenosine 3^1, 5^1-Monophosphate. *Science* 162:3861, 1484–1485, 27 December 1968.

Schlegel, J. U. Proposed Uses of Ascorbic Acid in Prevention of Bladder Carcinoma. *Annals of the New York Academy of Sciences* (Second Conference on Vitamin C) 258, 432–437, 1975.

——, Pipkin, G. E., Nishimura, E., and Shultz, G. N. The Role of Ascorbic Acid in the Prevention of Bladder Tumor Formation. *Journal of Urology* 103:2, 155–159, February 1970.

Shapley, D. Nitrosamines: Scientists on the Trail of Prime Suspect in Urban Cancer. *Science* 191:4224, 268–270, 23 January 1976.

Silverberg, E. Cancer Statistics, 1980. *Ca—A Cancer Journal for Clinicians* 30:1, 23–38, January–February 1980.

Spiegelhalder, B., Eisenbrand, G., and Pruessmann, R. Influence of Dietary Nitrate on Nitrite Content of Human Saliva: Possible Relevance to in Vivo Formation of N-Nitroso Compounds. *Food and Cosmetics Toxicology* 14:6, 545–548, December 1976.

Stone, I. *The Healing Factor: Vitamin C Against Disease.* 1972. New York, Grosset and Dunlap. Pp. 96–98.

Tannenbaum, S. R., Archer, M. C., Wishnok, J. S., Correa, P., Cuello, C., and Haenszel, W. Nitrate and the Etiology of Gastric Cancer. In Hiatt, H. H., Watson, J. D., and Watson, J. A., Editors. *Origins of Human Cancer.* 1977. New York, Cold Spring Harbor Laboratory. Pp. 1609–1625.

Tannenbaum, S. R., Fett, D., Young, V. R., Land, P. D., and Bruce, W. R. Nitrite and Nitrate Are Formed by Endogenous Synthesis in the Human Intestine. *Science* 200:4349, 1487–1489, 30 June 1978.

Tannenbaum, S. R., Weisman, M., and Fett, D. The Effect of Nitrate Intake on Nitrite Formation in Human Saliva. *Food and Cosmetics Toxicology* 14:6, 549–552, December 1976.

Walters, C. L. Vitamin C and Nitrosamine Formation. In Birch, G. G., and Parker, K. J. *Vitamin C: Recent Aspects of Its Physiological and Technological Importance.* 1974. New York, Wiley.

——, Carr, F. P. A., Dyke, C. S., Saxby, M. J., and Smith, P. L. R. Nitrite Sources and Nitrosamine Formation in Vitro and in Vivo. *Food and Cosmetics Toxicology* 17:5, 473–479, October 1979.

Wang, T., Kakizel, T., Dion, P., Furrer, R., Varghese, A. J., and Bruce, W. R. Volatile Nitrosamines in Normal Human Feces. *Nature*

276:5685, 280–281, 16 November 1978.

Washington (AP). Some Chemicals May Stave Off Cancer. *Birmingham News*, Tuesday, 15 July 1980.

Wassertheil-Smoller, S., Romney, S. L., Wylie-Rosett, J., Slagle, S., Miller, G., Lucido, D., Duttagupta, C., and Palah, P. Dietary Vitamin C and Uterine Cervical Dysplasia. *American Journal of Epidemiology* 114:5, 714–724, November 1981.

Weisburger, J. H. Vitamin C and Prevention of Nitrosamine Formation. *Lancet* 2:8038, 607, 17 September 1977.

——, Marquardt, H., Mower, H. F., Hirota, N., Mori, H., and Williams, G. Inhibition of Carcinogenesis: Vitamin C and the Prevention of Gastric Cancer. *Preventive Medicine* 9:3, 352–361, May 1980.

Wilson, C. W. M. Clinical Pharmacologic Aspects of Ascorbic Acid. *Annals of the New York Academy of Sciences* (Second Conference on Vitamin C) 258, 355–376, 1975.

Yonemoto, R. H., Chretian, P. B., and Fehniger, T. F. Enhanced Lymphocyte Blastogenesis by Oral Ascorbic Acid. *Proceedings of the American Association for Cancer Research and American Society of Clinical Oncology* 17: Abstract #C-206, 288, March 1976.

11. The "Tired Blood" Caper

Beaton, G. H. Epidemiology of Iron Deficiency. In Jacobs, A., and Worwood, M. *Iron in Biochemistry and Medicine.* 1974. New York, Academic Press. Pp. 477–528.

Cheraskin, E., Ringsdorf, W. M., Jr., and Medford, F. H. Daily Vitamin C Consumption and Fatigability. *Journal of the American Geriatrics Society* 24:3, 136–137, March 1976.

Cook, J. D., Finch, C. A., and Smith, N. J. Evaluation of Iron Status of a Population. *Blood* 48:3, 449–455, September 1976.

Cook, J. D., and Monsen, E. R. Vitamin C, the Common Cold, and Iron Absorption. *American Journal of Clinical Nutrition* 30:2, 235–241, February 1977.

Committee on Dietary Allowances. Food and Nutrition Board. *Recommended Dietary Allowances.* Ninth Revised Edition, 1980. Washington, D.C., National Academy of Sciences.

Cox, E. V. The Anemia of Scurvy. In Harris, R. S., Wool, I. G., and Loraine, J. A. *Vitamins and Hormones.* Volume 26. 1968. New York, Academic Press. Pp. 635–652.

Gaines, E. G., and Daniel, W. A. Dietary Iron Intake of Adolescents. *Journal of the American Dietetics Association* 65:3, 275–279, September 1974.

Kalchthaler, T., and Tan, M. E. R. Anemia in Institutionalized Elderly Patients. *Journal of the American Geriatrics Society* 28:3, 108–113, March 1980.

Kohrs, M.B., O'Neal, R., Preston, A., Eklund, D., and Abrahams, O. Nutritional Status of Elderly Residents in Missouri. *American Journal of Clinical Nutrition* 31:12, 2186–3297, December 1978.

Layrisse, M., Martinez-Torres, C., and Gonzales, M. Measurement of the Total Daily Iron Absorption by the Extrinsic Tag Model. *American Journal of Clinical Nutrition* 27:2, 152–162, February 1974.

McCurdy, P. R., and Dern, R. J. Some Therapeutic Implications of Ferrous Sulphate–Ascorbic Acid Mixtures. *American Journal of Clinical Nutrition* 21:4, 284–288, April 1968.

O'Brien, R. T. Ascorbic Acid Enhancement of Desferrioxamine-Induced Urinary Iron Excretion in Thalassemia Major. *Annals of the New York Academy of Sciences* 232, 221–225, 1974.

Rossander, L., Hallberg, L., and Björn-Rasmussen, E. Absorption of Iron from Breakfast Meals. *American Journal of Clinical Nutrition* 32:12, 2484–2489, December 1979.

Sayers, M. H., Lynch, S. R., Charlton, R. W., and Bothwell, T. H. Iron Absorption from Rice Meals Cooked with Fortified Salt Containing Ferrous Sulphate and Ascorbic Acid. *British Journal of Nutrition* 31:3, 367–375, May 1974.

Sayers, M. H., Lynch, S. R., Charlton, R. W., Bothwell, T. H., Walker, R. B., and Mayet, F. The Fortification of Common Salt with Ascorbic Acid and Iron. *British Journal of Haematology* 28:4, 483–495, December 1974.

Sayers, M. H., Lynch, S. R., Jacobs, P., Charlton, R. W., Bothwell, T. H., Walker, R. B., and Mayet, F. The Effects of Ascorbic Acid Supplementation on the Absorption of Iron in Maize, Wheat and Soya. *British Journal of Haematology* 24:2, 209–218, February 1973.

Stewart, C. P., and Guthrie, D. *Lind's Treatise on Scurvy.* 1953. Edinburgh, University Press.

United States Department of Health, Education, and Welfare. *Dietary Intake Source Data: United States, 1971–1974.* DHEW Publication No. (PHS) 72–1221. 1979. Hyattsville, Maryland, Office of Health Research, Statistics, and Technology.

Wapnick, A. A., Lynch, S. R., Charlton, R. W., Seftel, H. C., and Bothwell, T. H. The Effect of Ascorbic Acid Deficiency on Desferrioxamine-Induced Urinary Iron Excretion. *British Journal of Haematology* 17:6, 563–568, December 1969.

12. A "C" Full of Smiles

Aleo, J. J. Inhibition of Endotoxin-Induced Depression of Cellular Proliferation by Ascorbic Acid. *Proceedings of the Society for Experimental Biology and Medicine* 164:3, 248–251, July 1980.

———. Stimulation of Macromolecular Synthesis by Endotoxin-Treated 3T6 Fibroblasts. *Experienta* 36:5, 546–657, 1980.

Ascorbic Acid Regimen May Reduce Calculus. *Dental Times* 11:12, 1 and 5, 1968.

Cheraskin, E., and Ringsdorf, W. M., Jr. Biology of the Orthodontic Patient: II. Lingual Vitamin C Test Scores. *Angle Orthodontist* 39:4, 324–325, October 1969.

———. A Lingual Vitamin C Test: XIV. Relationship to Oral Calculus. *International Journal for Vitamin Research* 38:5, 531–537, 1968.

———. Biology of the Orthodontic Patient: I. Plasma Ascorbic Acid Levels. *Angle Orthodontist* 39:2, 137–138, April 1969.

———. Biology of the Orthodontic Patient. III. Relationship of Chronologic and Dental Age in Terms of Vitamin C State. *Angle Orthodontist* 42:1, 56–59, January 1972.

———. Vitamin C and Chronologic Versus Bone Age. *Journal of Oral Medicine* 28:3, 77–80, July/September 1973.

Cheraskin, E., Ringsdorf, W. M., Jr., Aspray, D. W., and Preskitt, D. A Lingual Vitamin C Test: XIII. Relationship to Oral Hygiene. *International Journal for Vitamin Research* 38:5, 524–530, 1968.

Cheraskin, E., Ringsdorf, W. M., Jr., and Medford, F. H. Tissue Tolerance to Orthodontic Banding: Two Studies in Multivitamin–Trace Mineral Versus Placebo Supplementation. *International Journal of Orthodontics* 17:4, 6–20, December 1979.

Cheraskin, E., Strother, E. W., and Speed, E. M. What Is Pyorrhea? *General Practice* 11:3, 69–73, March 1955.

Clark, J. W., Cheraskin, E., and Ringsdorf, W. M., Jr. An Ecologic Study of Oral Hygiene. *Journal of Periodontology-Periodontics* 40:8, 476–480, August 1969.

———. Diet and the Periodontal Patient. 1970. Springfield, Charles C. Thomas.

Cohen, D. W., Friedman, L. A., Shapiro, J., Kyle, G. C., and Franklin, S. Diabetes Mellitus and Periodontal Disease: Two-Year Longitudinal

Observations. Part I. *Journal of Periodontology* 41:12, 709–712, December 1970.

Cowan, A. The Influence of Vitamin C on the Periodontal Membrane Space—A Radiographic Study. *Irish Journal of Medical Science* 145:9, 273–284, September 1976.

El-Ashiry, G. M., Ringsdorf, W. M., Jr., and Cheraskin, E. Local and Systemic Influences in Periodontal Disease: II. Effect of Prophylaxis and Natural Versus Synthetic Vitamin C upon Gingivitis. *Journal of Periodontology* 35:3, 250–259, May/June 1964.

——. Local and Systemic Influences in Periodontal Disease: III. Effect of Prophylaxis and Natural Versus Synthetic Vitamin C upon Sulcus Depth. *New York Journal of Dentistry* 34:7, 254–262, August/September 1964.

——. Local and Systemic Influences in Periodontal Disease: IV. Effect of Prophylaxis and Natural Versus Synthetic Vitamin C Upon Clinical Tooth Mobility. *International Journal for Vitamin Research* 34:2, 202–218, 1964.

Goldhaber, P., and Rabadjija, L. Inhibition of Bone Resorption in Tissue Culture by Ascorbic Acid. *Journal of Dental Research* 55: Special Issue B, 220, February 1976.

Graber, T. M., and Swain, B. F. *Current Orthodontic Concepts and Techniques*. 1975. Second Edition. Philadelphia, W. B. Saunders.

Johansen, J. R., Flötra, L., and Gjermo, P. A Clinical Evaluation of the Effect of Ascoxal T on Plaque Formation and Gingivitis. *Acta Odontologica Scandinavica* 28:5, 661–677, November 1970.

Kutscher, A. H. Massive Vitamin C Therapy of Chronic Marginal Gingivitis. *New York State Dental Journal* 19:8, 422–424, October 1953.

Kyhos, E. D., Gordon, E. S., Kimble, M. S., and Sevringhaus, E. L. The Minimum Ascorbic Acid Need for Adults. *Journal of Nutrition* 27:3, 271–285, March 1944.

Linghorne, W. J., McIntosh, W. G., Tice, J. W., Tisdall, F. F., McCreary, J. F., Drake, T. G. H., Greaves, A. V., and Johnstone, W. M. The Relation of Ascorbic Acid Intake to Gingivitis. *Journal of the Canadian Dental Association* 12:2, 49–66, February 1946.

Mallek, H. M. An Investigation of the Role of Ascorbic Acid and Iron in the Etiology of Gingivitis in Humans. 1978. Ph.D. Dissertation, Massachusetts Institute of Technology.

McDonald, B. S. Gingivitis-Ascorbic Acid Deficiency in the Navajo. III. Dietary Aspects. *Journal of the American Dietetic Association* 43:4, 331–335, October 1963.

From the NIH. Primate Studies Indicate That Subclinical and Acute Vitamin C Deficiency May Lead to Periodontal Disease. *Journal of the American Medical Association* 246:7, 730, 14 August 1981.

O'Leary, T. J., Rudd, K. D., Crump, P. P., and Krause, R. E. The Effect of Ascorbic Acid Supplementation on Tooth Mobility. *Journal of Periodontology-Periodontics* 40:5, 284–286, May 1969.

Parfitt, G. J., and Hand, C. D. Reduced Plasma Ascorbic Acid Levels and Gingival Health. *Journal of Periodontology* 34:4, 347–351, July 1963.

Pierce, H. B., Newhall, C. A., Merrow, S. B., Lamden, M. P., Schweiker, C., and Laughlin, A. Ascorbic Acid Supplementation. I. Responses of Gum Tissue. *American Journal of Clinical Nutrition* 8:3, 353–362, May–June 1960.

Preventive Dentistry: The Pharmacist's Role. *Guidelines to Professional Pharmacy* 7:2, 1980.

Roff, F. S., and Glazebrook, A. J. The Therapeutic Use of Vitamin C in Gingivitis of Adolescents. *British Dental Journal* 68:4, 135–141, 15 February 1940.

Rudolph, C. E. An Evaluation of Root Resorption During Orthodontic Treatment. *Journal of Dental Research* 19:4, 367–371, August 1940.

Stamm, W. P., Macrae, T. F., and Yudkin, S. Incidence of Bleeding Gums Among R. A. F. Personnel and the Value of Ascorbic Acid in Treatment. *British Medical Journal* 2:4363, 239–241, 9 August 1944.

Stanton, G. Ascorbic Acid Regimen Can Reduce Calculus. *Dental Times* 11:12, 1, 5, December 1968.

Thomas, A. E., Busby, M. C., Jr., Ringsdorf, W. M., Jr., and Cheraskin, E. Gingival Hue and Orange Juice. *Journal of Dental Medicine* 18:4, 171–174, October 1963.

Tom, N. S. A Radiographic Study of Apical Root Resorption in Orthodontic Patients Taking Supplemental Time Release Vitamin C Capsules. Thesis. 1973. University of Detroit Dental Center.

Tully, W. J., and Cryer, B. S. *Orthodontic Treatment for the Adult.* 1969. Bristol, John Wright and Sons.

Vest, R. N., and Zion, H. *Prophylaxis and Vitamin C Therapy in Treating Gingivitis in Humans.* Unpublished data.

Vital and Health Statistics. *An Assessment of the Occlusion of the Teeth of Youths 12–17 Years. United States.* DHEW publication number (HRA) 77–1644. 1977. Washington, D.C. United States Department of Health, Education, and Welfare.

Vital and Health Statistics. *Basic Data on Dental Examination Findings of Persons 1–74 Years, United States, 1971–1974.* Series 11, Number 214. DHEW publication number (PHS) 79–1662. Washington, D.C.

United States Department of Health, Education, and Welfare.
Vital and Health Statistics. *Current Estimates from the Health Interview Survey: United States 1978.* Series 10, Number 130. 1979. Washington, D.C., United States Department of Health, Education, and Welfare.

Vital and Health Statistics. *Oral Hygiene in Adults. United States. 1960–1962.* 1966. Washington, D.C. United States Department of Health, Education, and Welfare.

Wasserman, E. The Effect of Ascorbic Acid Levels on Orthodontically Induced Tooth Mobility. Thesis. 1973. New York, New York University College of Dentistry.

13. Seeing with C

Bietti, G. B. Further Contributions on the Value of Osmotic Substances as Means to Reduce Intra-ocular Pressure. *Transactions of the Ophthalmological Society of Australia* 26:61–71, 1967.

Cheraskin, E., and Ringsdorf, W. M., Jr. *New Hope for Incurable Diseases.* 1971. Jericho, New York, Exposition Press.

Fishbein, S. L., and Goodstein, S. The Pressure Lowering Effect of Ascorbic Acid. *Annals of Ophthalmology* 4:6, 487–491, June 1972.

Lane, B. C. Evaluation of Intraocular Pressure with Daily, Sustained Closework Stimulus to Accommodation to Lowered Tissue Chromium and Dietary Deficiency of Ascorbic Acid (Vitamin C). Ph.D. dissertation, New York University. 1980.

Linner, E. Intraocular Pressure Regulation and Ascorbic Acid. *Acta Societatis, Medicorum, Upsaliensis* 69:5–6, 225–232, 1964.

———. The Pressure Lowering Effect of Ascorbic Acid in Ocular Hypertension. *Acta Ophthalmologica* 47:3, 685–689, 1969.

Shen, T.-M., and Yü, M.-C. Clinical Evaluation of Glycerin-Sodium Ascorbate Solution in Lowering Intraocular Pressure. *Chinese Medical Journal* 1:1–6, 64–68, January 1975.

Stocker, F. W. New Ways of Influencing the Intraocular Pressure. *New York State Journal of Medicine* 49:1, 58–63, January 1949.

Virno, M., Bucci, M. G., Pecori-Giraldi, J., and Missiroli, A. Oral Treatment of Glaucoma with Vitamin C. *Eye, Ear, Nose and Throat Monthly* 46:12, 1502–1508, December 1967.

14. It's *Not* All in Your Mind!

Bonham, G. S. *Use Habits of Cigarettes, Coffee, Aspirin and Sleeping Pills, United States 1976.* Vital and Health Statistics Series 10, Data from the National Health Survey: 131, DHEW publication (PHS) 80–1559.

Brin, M. Example of Behavioral Changes in Marginal Vitamin Deficiency in the Rat and Man. In Brozek, Josef, editor. *Behavioral Effects of Energy and Protein Deficits.* Proceedings International Nutrition Conference, NIH Publication 79-1906, August 1979.

Cheraskin, E., and Ringsdorf, W. M., Jr. The Mental Illness Proneness Profile. *Alabama Journal of Medical Science* 10:1, 32–45, January 1973.

Dupuy, H. J., Engel, A., Devine, B. K., Scanlon, J., and Overec, L. *Selected Symptoms of Psychologic Distress, United States 1970.* Vital and Health Statistics: Series 11, Data from the National Health Survey: 37, DHEW publication (PHS) 1000.

Eddy, T. P. The Problem of Retaining Vitamins in Hospital Food. In Exton-Smith, A. N., and Scott, D. L., editors. *Vitamins in the Elderly.* 1968. Bristol, England, John Wright and Sons. Pp. 86–92.

Hodges, R. E., Baker, E. M., Hood, J., Sauberlich, H. E., and March, S. C. Experimental Scurvy in Man. *American Journal of Clinical Nutrition* 22:5, 535–548, May 1969.

Jancar, J. Gradual Withdrawal of Tranquilizers with the Help of Ascorbic Acid. *British Journal of Psychiatry* 117:537, 238–239, August 1970.

Kubala, A. L., and Katz, M. W. Nutritional Factors in Psychological Test Behavior. *Journal of Genetic Psychology* 96, 343–352, Second Half, 1960.

Milner, G. Ascorbic Acid in Chronic Psychiatric Patients—A Controlled Trial. *British Journal of Psychiatry* 109:459, 294–299, March 1963.

Naylor, G. J. New Approaches to the Treatment of Manic-Depressive Illness. *Neuropharmacology* 19:12, 1233–1234, December 1980.

Osmond, H., and Hoffer, A. Naturally Occurring Endogenous Major and Minor Tranquilizers. *Journal of Orthomolecular Psychiatry* 9:3, 198–206, Third Quarter 1980.

Physician's Desk Reference (PDR). Thirty-Fourth Edition, 1980. Charles E. Baker, Jr.

Sayetta, R. B. *Basic Data on Depressive Symptomatology, United States 1974–75.* Vital and Health Statistics: Series 11, Data from the National

Health Survey: 216, DHEW publication number (PHS) 80-1666.

Sedlmair, M., and Sisley, E. L. Mural Group: Integration of Projective Drawings with Standard Verbal Group Therapy Practices. *Psychological Reports* 31, 475–481, 1972.

Sisley, E. L. Differential Perception of Kinget's Drawing-Completion Stimuli. *Perceptual and Motor Skills* 35, 491–494, 1972.

———. The Meaning of Drawing-Completion Stimuli: New Guidelines for Projective Interpretation. *Journal of Personality Assessment* 37, 64–68, 1973.

———. The Breakdown of the American Image: Comparison of Stereotypes Held by College Students Over Four Decades. *Psychological Reports* 27, 779–786, 1970.

Spector, R., and Lorenzo, A. V. Ascorbic Acid Homeostasis in the Central Nervous System. *American Journal of Physiology* 225:4, 757–763, October 1973.

———. Specificity of Ascorbic Acid Transport System of the Central Nervous System. *American Journal of Physiology* 226:6, 1468–1473, June 1974.

15. Addiction Plus Vitamin C Equals No Addiction

Bejerot, N. *Addiction: An Artificially Induced Drive.* 1972. Springfield, Charles C. Thomas.

Cameron, E., and Baird, G. M. Ascorbic Acid and Dependence on Opiates in Patients with Advanced and Disseminated Cancer. *Journal of the International Research Communications* 1:6, 38, August 1973.

Free, V., and Sanders, P. The Use of Ascorbic Acid and Mineral Supplements in the Detoxification of Narcotic Addicts. *Journal of Orthomolecular Psychiatry* 7:4, 264–270, 1978.

Jancar, J. Gradual Withdrawal of Tranquilizers with the Help of Ascorbic Acid. *British Journal of Psychiatry* 117:537, 238–239, August 1970.

Libby, A. F., and Stone, I. The Hypoascorbemia-kwashiorkor Approach to Drug Addiction Therapy: A Pilot Study. *Journal of Orthomolecular Psychiatry* 6:4, 300–308, Fourth Quarter 1977.

Scher, J., Rice, H., Kim, S., DiCamelli, R., and O'Conner, H. Massive Vitamin C as an Adjunct in Methadone Maintenance and Detoxification. *Journal of Orthomolecular Psychiatry* 5:3, 191–198, Third Quarter 1976.

Walker, K. *The Story of Medicine.* 1955. New York, Oxford University Press.

16. Plugging in More Connections

Cheraskin, E., Ringsdorf, W. M., Jr., Medford, F. H., and Hicks, B. S. Relationship of Vitamin C and Skin Symptoms and Signs. *Journal of the Canadian Chiropractic Association* 22:3, 97–98, October 1978.

———. The Relationship of Vitamin C Intake and the Total White Cell Count. *Nutritional Perspectives* 1:2, 34–36, April 1978.

Cotlier, E., and Duwelius, A. Effect of Ascorbic Acid on Hexosaminidase Activity. *New England Journal of Medicine* 285:7, 409, 12 August 1971.

Cousins, N. Anatomy of an Illness (as Perceived by the Patient). *New England Journal of Medicine* 295:26, 1458–1463, 23 December 1976.

———. *Anatomy of an Illness.* 1979. New York, W. W. Norton.

Desnick, R. J., and Goldberg, J. D. Tay-Sachs Disease: Prospects for Therapeutic Intervention. In Kabach, M. M. *Tay-Sachs Disease: Screening and Prevention.* 1977. New York, Alan R. Liss.

Eaton, J. W., Kolpin, C. F., and Kjellstrand, C.-M. Chlorinated Urban Water. A Cause of Dialysis-Induced Hemolytic Anemia. *Science* 181:4098, 463–464, 3 August 1973.

Greenwood, J., Jr. On Osteoarthritis, the "Wear and Tear" Disease . . . Can Vitamin C Help? *Executive Health* 16:7, April 1980.

Hansky, J., and Allmand, F. Gastro-Intestinal Bleeding: The Role of Vitamin C. *Australian Annals of Medicine* 18:3, 248–250, August 1969.

Hormones and Impotence. *Science News* 117:9, 136, 1 March 1980.

Igarashi, M. Augmentative Effect of Ascorbic Acid upon Induction of Human Ovulation in Clomiphene-Ineffective Anovulatory Women. *International Journal of Fertility* 22:3, 168–173, 1977.

Inglemark, B. E. Cited in Evans, F. G. *Biochemical Studies of the Musculoskeletal System.* 1961. Springfield, Charles C. Thomas.

Kaback, M. M. *Tay-Sachs Disease: Screening and Prevention.* 1977. New York, Alan R. Liss, Inc.

Lewin, S. Evaluation of Potential Effects of High Intake of Ascorbic Acid. *Comparative Biochemistry and Physiology* 47:3, 681–695, 15 March 1974.

Lind, J. A *Treatise of the Scurvy.* First Edition. 1753. Edinburgh, Sands, Murray and Cochran.

Mankin, H. J. Cited in Greenwood, J., Jr. On Osteoarthritis, the "Wear and Tear" Disease . . . Can Vitamin C Help? *Executive Health* 16:7, April 1980.

Miller, J. Z., Nance, W. E., Norton, J. A., Wolen, R. L., Griffith, R. S., and Rose, R. J. Therapeutic Effect of Vitamin C. A Co-Twin Control

Study. *Journal of the American Medical Association* 237:3, 248–251, 17 January 1977.

Milner, J. E. Ascorbic Acid in the Prevention of Chromium Dermatitis. *Journal of Occupational Medicine* 22:1, 51–52, January 1980.

Okada, S., and O'Brien, J. S. Tay-Sachs Disease: Generalized Absence of a Beta-D-N-Acetylhexosaminidase Component. *Science* 165:3894, 698–700, 15 August 1969.

Robinson, A. B., Catchpool, J. R., and Pauling L. Decreased White Blood Cell Count in People Who Supplement Their Diet with L-Ascorbic Acid. *International Research Communication Systems* 3, 259, 1975.

Robinson, D., and Stirling, J. L. N-Acetyl-Beta-Glucosaminidases in Human Spleen. *Biochemical Journal* 107:3, 321–327, April 1968.

Samitz, M. H. Ascorbic Acid in the Prevention and Treatment of Toxic Effects of Chromates. *Acta Dermatovenereologica* 50:1, 59–64, 1970.

Sandhoff, K., Andreae, U., and Jatzkewitz, H. Deficient Hexosaminidase Activity in an Exceptional Case of Tay-Sachs Disease with Additional Storage of Kidney Globoside in Visceral Organs. *Life Sciences* 7:6, 283–288, 15 March 1968.

Schorah, C. J., Scott, D. L., Newill, A., and Morgan, D. B. Clinical Effects of Vitamin C in Elderly Inpatients with Low Blood-Vitamin-C Levels. *Lancet* 1:8113, 403–405, 24 February 1979.

Spark, R. F., White, R. A., and Connolly, P. B. Impotence Is Not Always Psychogenic: Newer Insights into Hypothalamic-Pituitary-Gonadal Dysfunction. *Journal of the American Medical Association* 243:8, 750–755, 22/29 February 1980.

Wilson, T. S., Datta, S. B., Murrell, J. S., and Andrews, C. T. Relation of Vitamin C Levels to Mortality in a Geriatric Hospital: A Study of the Effect of Vitamin C Administration. *Age & Ageing* 2:3, 163–171, 1973.

17. How Much C Do I Have?

Abramson, J. H., Slome, C., and Kosovsky, C. Food Frequency Interview as an Epidemiological Tool. *American Journal of Public Health* 53:7, 1093–1101, July 1963.

Adams, C. F. *Nutritive Value of American Foods*. Agriculture Handbook No. 456. 1975. Agricultural Research Service, United States Department of Agriculture. Washington, D.C. United States Government Printing Office.

Burch, H. B. Methods for Detecting and Evaluating Ascorbic Acid Deficiency in Man and Animals. *Annals of the New York Academy of Sciences* 92:1, 268–276, 21 April 1961.

Butterworth, C. E., Jr. *Nutrition Assessment of Ambulatory Patients.* Vitamin Nutrition Issues. 1979. Nutley, New Jersey, Hoffman-La Roche. Pp. 25–28.

Cameron, E., and Pauling, L. *Cancer and Vitamin C.* 1979. New York, W. W. Norton. P. 106.

Chalmers, F. W., Clayton, M. M., Gates, L. O., Tucker, R. E., Wertz, A. W., Young, C. M., and Foster, W. D. The Dietary Record—How Many and Which Days? *Journal of the American Dietetic Association* 28:8, 711–717, August 1952.

Cheraskin, E., and Ringsdorf, W. M., Jr. A Lingual Vitamin C Test: VII. Relationship of Nonfasting Serum Cholesterol and Vitamin C State. *International Journal for Vitamin Research* 38:3/4, 415–420, 1968.

———. A Lingual Vitamin C Test: XIX. Normal versus Physiologic Range. *Journal of the Ontario Dental Association* 47:10, 239–241, October 1970.

Cheraskin, E., Ringsdorf, W. M., Jr., Hicks, B. S., and Romano, D. M. The Prevention of Oral Disease. *Journal of the International Academy of Preventive Medicine* 2:1, 22–52, First Quarter 1975.

Christakis, G. Nutritional Assessment in Health Programs. *American Journal of Public Health* 63: Supplement 1, 11–18, November 1973.

Church, C. F. *Bowes and Church Food Values of Portions Commonly Used.* 1966. Tenth Edition. Philadelphia, J. B. Lippincott.

Denson, K. W., and Bowers, E. F. The Determination of Ascorbic Acid in White Blood Cells. *Clinical Science* 21:2, 157–162, October 1961.

Dunbar, J. B., Cheraskin, E., and Flynn, F. H. The Intradermal Ascorbic Test: Part II. A Review of Human Studies. *Journal of Dental Medicine* 13:1, 19–40, January 1958.

Evans, S. N., and Gormican, A. The Computer in Retrieving Dietary History Data. I. Designing and Evaluating a Computerized Diabetic Dietary History. *Journal of the American Dietetic Association* 63:4, 397–402, October 1973.

Giza, T., and Weclawowicz, J. Perlingual Method for Evaluating the Vitamin C Content of the Body: A Rapid Diagnostic Test for Vitamin C Undernutrition. *International Review of Vitamin Research* 30:3, 327–332, 1960.

Hsu, N., and Gormican, A. The Computer in Retrieving Dietary History Data. II. Retrieving Information by Summary Generation. *Journal of the American Dietetic Association* 63:4, 402–407, October 1973.

Loh, H. S. The Relationship Between Dietary Ascorbic Acid Intake and

Buffy Coat and Plasma Ascorbic Acid Concentrations at Different Ages. *International Journal for Vitamin and Nutrition Research* 42:1, 80–85, 1972.

Marr, J. W. Dietary Survey Methods: Individual and Group Aspects. *Proceedings of the Royal Society of Medicine* 66:7, 639–641, July 1973.

Mason, M., Wenberg, B. G., and Welsch, P. K. *The Dynamics of Clinical Dietetics.* 1977. New York, Wiley. Pp. 114–140.

Race, G. J., and White, M. G. *Basic Urinalysis.* 1979. New York, Harper & Row.

Ringsdorf, W. M., Jr., and Cheraskin, E. The Lingual Ascorbic Acid Test. *Quintessence International* 12:1707, 81–85, December 1978.

Sauberlich, H. E. Vitamin C Status: Methods and Findings. *Annals of the New York Academy of Sciences* 258, 438–450, 30 September 1975.

Sebrell, W. H., and Harris, R. S. *The Vitamins: Chemistry, Physiology, Pathology, Methods.* Second Edition. Volume I. 1967. New York, Academic Press.

Servaas, C., and Mathews, W. *The Vitamin C Cookbook.* 1975. Garden City, New York, Doubleday and Company, Inc.

Watt, B. K., and Merrill, A. L. *Composition of Foods: Raw, Processed, Prepared.* Agriculture Handbook No. 8. 1975. Consumer and Food Economics Institute, Agricultural Research Service, United States Department of Agriculture. Washington, D.C., United States Government Printing Office.

Widdowson, E. M., and McCance, R. A. Food Tables: Their Scope and Limitations. *Lancet* 1:6234, 230–232, 20 February 1943.

Witschi, J., Porter, D., Vogel, S., Buxbaum, R., State, F. J., and Slack, W. A Computer-Based Dietary Counseling System. *Journal of the American Dietetic Association* 69:4, 385–390, October 1976.

Yew, M.-L. S., and Lo, Y. Levels of Optimal Vitamin C Intake in Individuals as Estimated by the Lingual Tests. *Proceedings of the Society for Experimental Medicine and Surgery* 144:2, 626–627, November 1973.

Yung, S., Mayersohn, M., and Robinson, J. B. Ascorbic Acid Absorption in Man: Influence of Divided Dose and Food. *Life Sciences* 28:22, 2505–2511, 1981.

18. How Much C Do I Need?

Cheraskin, E., Ringsdorf, W. M., Jr., and Medford, F. H. The "Ideal" Daily Vitamin C Intake. *Journal of the Medical Association of the State of Alabama* 46:12, 39–40, June 1977.

Fabry, P., Fodor, J., Hejl, Z., Braun, T., and Zvolankova, K. The Frequency of Meals: Its Relation to Overweight, Hypercholesterolaemia, and Decreased Glucose Tolerance. *Lancet* 2:7360, 614–615, 19 September 1964.

Food and Nutrition Board. *Recommended Dietary Allowances.* Ninth Revised Edition, 1979. 1980, Washington, D.C., National Academy of Sciences.

Hawkins, D., and Pauling, L. *Orthomolecular Psychiatry.* 1973. San Francisco, W. H. Freeman.

Hodges, R. E., Hood, J., Canham, J. E., Sauberlich, H. E., and Baker, E. M. Clinical Manifestations of Ascorbic Acid Deficiency in Man. *American Journal of Clinical Nutrition* 24:4, 432–443, April 1971.

How Vitamin C Really Works . . . or Does It? *Nutrition Today* 14:5, 6–7, 15–19, September/October 1979.

Irwin, M. I., and Hutchins, B. K. A Conspectus of Research on Vitamin C Requirements of Man. *Journal of Nutrition* 106:6, 823–879, June 1976.

Klenner, F. R. Significance of High Daily Intake of Ascorbic Acid in Preventive Medicine. In Williams, R. J., and Kalita, D. K. *A Physician's Handbook on Orthomolecular Medicine.* 1977. New York, Pergamon Press. Pp. 51–59.

Pauling, L. Are Recommended Daily Allowances for Vitamin C Adequate? *Proceedings of the National Academy of Sciences* 71:11, 4442–4446, November 1974.

———. For the Best of Health—How Much Vitamin C Do You Need? *Executive Health* 12:3, December 1975.

Physicians' Desk Reference (PDR): Nonprescription Drugs. First Edition. 1980. Charles E. Baker, Jr.

Physicians' Desk Reference (PDR). Thirty-Fourth Edition. 1980. Charles E. Baker, Jr.

The Recommended Dietary Allowances. RDAs Part I. The New Recommended Dietary Allowances. *Nutrition Today* 14:5, 10–14, September/October 1979.

Stone, I. *The Healing Factor: Vitamin C Against Disease.* 1972. New York, Grosset and Dunlap.

Subcommittee on Laboratory Animal Nutrition. *Nutrient Requirements of Laboratory Animals.* Second Edition. 1972. Washington, D. C., National Academy of Sciences.

Vital and Health Statistics. *Health Characteristics of Low-Income Persons.* Series 10, Number 74. DHEW publication number (HSM) 73–1500. United States Department of Health, Education, and Welfare. July 1972.

Vital and Health Statistics. *Prevalence of Chronic Conditions of the Genitourinary, Nervous, Endocrine, Metabolic, and Blood and Blood-Forming Systems and of Other Selected Chronic Conditions.* Series 10, Number 109. DHEW publication number (HRA) 77–1536. United States Department of Health, Education, and Welfare. March 1977.

Vital and Health Statistics. *Skin Conditions and Related Need for Medical Care Among Persons 1–74 Years, United States, 1971–1974.* Series 11, Number 212. DHEW publication number (PHS) 79–1660. United States Department of Health, Education, and Welfare. November 1978.

Vital and Health Statistics. *Use Habits Among Adults of Cigarettes, Coffee, Aspirin, and Sleeping Pills.* Series 10, Number 131, DHEW publication number (PHS) 80–1559. United States Department of Health, Education, and Welfare. October 1979.

Williams, R. *Biochemical Individuality: The Basis for the Genetrophic Concept.* 1969. Austin, Texas, University of Texas Press.

——. *You Are Extraordinary.* 1967. New York, Random House.

Yew, M. S. "Recommended Daily Allowances" for Vitamin C. *Proceedings of the National Academy of Sciences* 70:969–972, 1973.

19. Can Vitamin C Hurt You?

Afroz, M., Bhothinard, B., Etzkorn, J. R., Horenstein, S., and McGarry, J. D. Vitamins C and B_{12}. *Journal of the American Medical Association* 232:3, 246, 21 April 1975.

Aldridge, H. Vitamin Megadoses Are Harmful, Either Insidiously or Dramatically, and Unnecessary, Physician Says. *Arkansas Gazette,* Little Rock, Arkansas, Thursday, 13 November 1975.

Alleva, F. R., Alleva, J. J., and Balazs, T. Effect of Large Daily Doses of Ascorbic Acid on Pregnancy in Guinea Pigs, Rats and Hamsters. *Toxicology and Applied Pharmacology* 35:2, 393–395, February 1976.

Barness, L. A. Safety Considerations with High Ascorbic Acid Dosage. *Annals of the New York Academy of Sciences* 258: Second Conference on Vitamin C, 523–527, 1975.

Barrows, G. H., Burton, R. M., Jarrett, D. D., Russell, G. G., Alford, M. D., and Songster, C. L. Immunochemical Detection of Human Blood in Feces. *American Journal of Clinical Pathology* 69:3, 342–346, March 1978.

Brandt, R., Colyer, K. E., and Banks, W. C., Jr. A Simple Method to Prevent Vitamin C Interference with Urinary Glucose Determinations. *Clinica Chemica Acta* 51:1, 103–104, 28 February 1974.

Briggs, M. H. Effects of Vitamin C on Bilirubin. *Medical Journal of Australia* 2:14, 542–543, 5 October 1974.

———. Fertility and High-Dose Vitamin C. *Lancet* 2:7837, 1083, 10 November 1973.

———. More Vitamin C. *Medical Journal of Australia* 1:18, 722–723, 4 May 1974.

———. Side-Effects of Vitamin C. *Lancet* 2:7843, 1439, 22 December 1973.

———. Vitamin C and Infertility. *Lancet* 2:7830, 677–678, 22 September 1973.

Briggs, M. H., Garcia-Webb, P., and Davies, P. Urinary Oxalate and Vitamin C Supplements. *Lancet* 2:7822, 201, 28 July 1973.

Briggs, M. H., and Johnson, J. Dangers of Excess Vitamin C. *Medical Journal of Australia* 2:1, 48–49, 7 July 1973.

Campbell, G. D., Jr., Steinberg, M. H., and Bower, J. D. Ascorbic Acid-Induced Hemolysis in G-6-PD Deficiency. *Annals of Internal Medicine* 82:6, 810, June 1975.

Churchill, D., Bryant, D. Fodor, G., and Gault, M. H. Drinking Water Hardness and Urolithiasis. *Annals of Internal Medicine* 88:4, 513–514, April 1978.

Corbetti, B. Big Doses of Vitamin C Branded More Harm Than Help. San Diego *Evening Tribune*, 7 December 1974.

DeCosse, J. J., Adams, M. B., Kuzma, J. F., LoGerfo, P., and Condon, R. E. Effect of Ascorbic Acid on Rectal Polyps of Patients with Familial Polyposis. *Surgery* 78:5, 608–612, November 1975.

DeRitter, E., Magid, L., Osadca, M., and Rubin, S. H. Effect of Silica Gel on Stability and Biological Availability of Ascorbic Acid. *Journal of Pharmaceutical Sciences* 59:2, 229–232, February 1970.

Diehl, H. S. Vitamin C for Colds. *American Journal of Public Health* 61:4, 646–651, April 1971.

Earnest, D. L. Perspectives on Incidence, Etiology, and Treatment of Enteric Hyperoxaluria. *American Journal of Clinical Nutrition* 30:1, 72–75, January 1977.

Frohberg, H., Gleich, J., and Kieser, H. Reproduktion Stoxikologische Studien mit Ascorbinsaure an Mausen und Ratten. *Arzneim Forsch* 23:8, 1081–1082, August 1973.

Gershoff, S. N., and Prien, E. L. Effect of Daily MgO and Vitamin B_6 Administration to Patients with Recurring Calcium Oxalate Kidney Stones. *American Journal of Clinical Nutrition* 20:5, 393–399, May 1967.

Guthrie, H. A., and Carter, J. The Issue of Supplementation. Presentation Summaries of Vitamin Nutrition Issues, October 26–28, 1979, Boca Raton, Florida. Sponsored by Vitamin Nutrition Information Service of Hoffman-La Roche, Inc., Nutley, New Jersey.

Hagler, L., and Herman, R. H. Oxalate Metabolism. II. *American Journal of Clinical Nutrition* 26:8, 882–889, August 1973.

Hanck, A. B. Blood Coagulation in Man During a Three Week Daily 4gL(+)–Ascorbic Acid Administration. *Blut* (München) 30:1, 47–50, January 1975.

———. Different Urine Parameters in Healthy Human Subjects During Intake of 4gL(+)–Ascorbic Acid. *International Journal for Vitamin and Nutrition Research* 44:3, 302–308, 1974.

———. Effect of 1000 mg. Per Day of Vitamin C on Renal Excretion of Some Electrolytes in Urine of Healthy Men. *International Journal for Vitamin and Nutrition Research* 43:1, 34–41, 1973.

———. The Influence on Vitamin Requirement of 4gL(+)–Ascorbic Acid Per Day in Healthy Humans. *International Journal for Vitamin and Nutrition Research* 44:1, 107–115, 1974.

Herbert, V. Facts and Fictions about Megavitamin Therapy. *Resident and Staff Physician* 24:13, 43–50, December 1978.

———. Megavitamin Therapy: Facts and Fictions. *Food and Nutrition News* 47:4, 3–4, March/April 1976.

———, and Jacob, E. Destruction of Vitamin B_{12} by Ascorbic Acid. *Journal of the American Medical Association* 230:2, 241–242, 14 October 1974.

———, ———, Wong, K. T. J., Scott, J., and Pfeffer, R. D. Low Serum Vitamin B_{12} Levels in Patients Receiving Ascorbic Acid in Megadoses; Studies Concerning the Effect of Ascorbate on Radioisotope Vitamin B_{12} Assay. *American Journal of Clinical Nutrition* 31:2, 253–258, February 1978.

Hines, J. D. Ascorbic Acid and Vitamin B_{12} Deficiency. *Journal of the*

American Medical Association (Letters) 234:1, 24, 6 October 1975.

Hoffer, A. Ascorbic Acid and Toxicity. *New England Journal of Medicine* 285:11, 635–636, 9 September 1971.

——. Vitamin C and Infertility. *Lancet* 2:7838, 1146, 17 November 1973.

Hogenkamp, H. P. C. The Interaction Between Vitamin B_{12} and Vitamin C. *The American Journal of Clinical Nutrition* 33:1, 1–3, January 1980.

Hornig, D., Weiser, H., Weber, F., and Wiss, O. Effect of Massive Doses of Ascorbic Acid on Its Catabolism in Guinea Pigs. *International Journal for Vitamin and Nutrition Research* 43:1, 28–33, 1973.

Horrobin, D. F. D.V.T. After Vitamin C? *Lancet* 2:7824, 317, 11 August 1973.

Igarashi, M. Augmentative Effect of Ascorbic Acid upon Induction of Human Ovulation in Clomiphene-Ineffective Anovulatory Women. *International Journal of Fertility* 22:3, 168–173, 1977.

Jaffe, R. M., Kasten, B., Young, D. S., and MacLowery, J. D. False-Negative Stool Occult Blood Tests Caused by Ingestion of Ascorbic Acid (Vitamin C). *Annals of Internal Medicine* 83:6, 824–826, December 1975.

Jaffe, R. M., Lawrence, L., Schmid, A., and MacLowry, J. D. Inhibition by Ascorbic Acid (Vitamin C) of Chemical Detection of Blood in Urine. *American Journal of Clinical Pathology* 72:3, 468–470, September 1979.

Jaffe, R. M., and Zierdt, W. A New Occult Blood Test Not Subject to False-Negative Results from Reducing Substances. *Journal of Laboratory and Clinical Medicine* 93:5, 879–886, May 1979.

Katz, S. M., and DiSilvio, T. V. Ascorbic Acid Effects on Serum Glucose Values. *Journal of the American Medical Association* 224:5, 628, 30 April 1973.

Klenner, F. R. Observations on the Dose and Administration of Ascorbic Acid When Employed Beyond the Range of a Vitamin in Human Pathology. *Journal of Applied Nutrition* 23:3–4, 61–88, Winter 1971.

Korner, W. F., and Weber, F. Tolerance for High Doses of Ascorbic Acid. *International Journal for Vitamin and Nutrition Research* 42:4, 528–544, 1972.

Lamden, M. P. Dangers of Massive Vitamin C Intake. *New England Journal of Medicine* 284:6, 336–337, 11 February 1971.

——, and Chrystowski, G. A. Urinary Oxalate Excretion by Man Following Ascorbic Acid Ingestion. *Proceedings of the Society for Experimental Biology and Medicine* 85:1, 190–192, January 1954.

Lewin, S. Recent Advances in the Molecular Biology of Vitamin C. In Birch, G. G., and Parker, K. J., Editors. *Vitamin C: Recent Aspects of Its Physiological and Technological Importance.* 1974. New York, Wiley. Pp. 221–251.

——. *Vitamin C: Its Molecular Biology and Medical Potential.* 1976. New York, Academic Press. Pp. 166–168.

Marcus, M., Prabhudesai, M., and Wassef, S. Stability of Vitamin B_{12} in the Presence of Ascorbic Acid in Food and Serum: Restoration by Cyanide of Apparent Loss. *American Journal of Clinical Nutrition* 33:1, 137–143, January 1980.

Mayson, J. S., Schumaker, O., and Nakamura, R. M. False-Negative Tests for Urinary Glucose in the Presence of Ascorbic Acid. *American Journal of Clinical Pathology* 58:3, 297–299, September 1972.

Nahata, M. C., and McLeod, D. C. Noneffect of Oral Ascorbic Acid on Urinary Copper Reduction Glucose Test. *Diabetes Care* 1:1, 34–35, January/February 1978.

Newmark, H. L., Scheiner, J., Marcus, M., and Prabhudesai, M. Stability of Vitamin B_{12} in the Presence of Ascorbic Acid. *American Journal of Clinical Nutrition* 29:6, 645–649, June 1976.

Nobile, S. R. Dangers of Excess Vitamin C. *Medical Journal of Australia* 2:6, 296, 11 August 1973.

Norkus, E. P., and Rosso, P. Changes in Ascorbic Acid Metabolism Following High Maternal Intake of This Vitamin in the Pregnant Guinea Pig. *Annals of the New York Academy of Sciences* 258: Second Conference on Vitamin C, 401–409, 1975.

Physician's Desk Reference (PDR). Published annually by Charles E. Baker, Jr.

Poser, E. Large Ascorbic Acid Intake. *New England Journal of Medicine* 287:8, 412, 24 August 1972.

Prauer, H. W. Vitamin C and Tests for Diabetes. *New England Journal of Medicine* 284:23, 1328, 10 June 1971.

Prien, E. L., Sr., and Gershoff, S. F. Magnesium Oxide-Pyridoxine Therapy for Recurrent Calcium Oxalate Calculi. *Journal of Urology* 112:4, 509–512, October 1974.

Rhead, W. J. Determinants of Ascorbic Acid Levels. *New England Journal of Medicine* 290:18, 1024–1028, 2 May 1974.

——, and Schrauzer, G. N. Risks of Long-Term Ascorbic Acid Overdosage. *Nutrition Reviews* 29:11, 262–263, November 1971.

Rhee, K. S., and Stubbs, A. C. Health Food Users in Two Texas Cities. Nutritional and Socioeconomic Implications. *Journal of the American*

Dietetic Association 68:6, 542–545, June 1976.

Ringsdorf, W. M., Jr., and Cheraskin, E. Nutritional Aspects of Urolithiasis. *Southern Medical Journal* 74:1, 41–43, 46, January 1981.

Roth, D. A., and Breitenfield, R. V. Vitamin C and Oxalate Stones. *Journal of the American Medical Association* 237:8, 768, 21 February 1977.

Scarlett, J. A., Zeidler, A., Rochman, H., and Rubenstein, A. Acute Effect of Ascorbic Acid Infusion on Carbohydrate Tolerance. *American Journal of Clinical Nutrition* 29:12, 1339–1342, December 1976.

Schrauzer, G. N. Vitamin C: Conservative Human Requirements and Aspects of Overdosage. In *International Review of Biochemistry, Biochemistry of Nutrition IA*. Volume 27. Neuberger, A., and Jukes, T. H., Editors. 1979. Baltimore, University Park Press, Pp. 167–187.

——, and Rhead, W. J. Ascorbic Acid Abuse: Effects of Long-Term Ingestion of Excessive Amounts on Blood Levels and Urinary Excretion. *International Journal for Vitamin and Nutrition Research* 43:2, 201–211, 1973.

Siegel, C., Barker, B., and Kunstadter, M. Conditioned Oral Scurvy Due to Megavitamin C Withdrawal. *Journal of Periodontology* 53:7, 453–455, July 1982.

Smith, L. H. Medical Evaluation of Urolithiasis: Etiologic Aspects and Diagnostic Evaluation. *Urological Clinics of North America* 1:2, 241–260, June 1974.

——, Van Den Berg, C. J., and Wilson, D. M. Nutrition and Urolithiasis. *New England Journal of Medicine* 298:2, 87–89, 12 January 1978.

Spiegel, H. E., and Pinili, E. Effect of Vitamin C on SGOT, SGPT, LDH, and Bilirubin. *Medical Journal of Australia* 2:7, 265–266, 17 August 1974.

Stauffer, J. O. Hyperoxaluria and Calcium Oxalate Nephrolithiasis After Jejunoileal Bypass. *American Journal of Clinical Nutrition* 30:1, 64–71, January 1977.

Stein, H. B., Hasan, A., and Fox, I. H. Ascorbic Acid-Induced Uricosuria. *Annals of Internal Medicine* 84:4, 385–388, April 1976.

Stone, I. The Genesis of Medical Myths. *Journal of Orthomolecular Psychiatry* 5:3, 163–168, Third Quarter, 1976.

Thom, J. A., Morris, J. E., Bishop, A., and Blacklock, N. J. The Influence of Refined Carbohydrate on Urinary Calcium Excretion. *British Journal of Urology* 50:7, 459–464, December 1978.

Tiselius, H. G. Excretion of 4-Pyridoxic Acid and Oxalic Acid in Patients with Urinary Calculi. *Investigative Urology* 15:1, 5–8, July 1977.

Vitamin Nutrition Information Service, Hoffmann-La Roche. Presentation Summaries, Vitamin Nutrition Issues, October 26–28, 1979, Boca Raton, Florida.

von Hilsheimer, G., Philpott, W., Milner, P. M., and Tucker, T. Ascorbic Acid Metabolism in a Population of Adolescent Psychiatric Patients. *Journal of Orthomolecular Psychiatry* 5:1, 43–44, First Quarter, 1976.

Wilson, C. W. M. Vitamin C: Tissue Metabolism, Over-Saturation, Desaturation, and Compensation. In Birch, G. G., and Parker, K. J., Editors. *Vitamin C: Recent Aspects of Its Physiological and Technological Importance.* 1974. New York, Wiley. Pp. 203–220.

——, and Loh, H. S. Vitamin C and Fertility. *Lancet* 2:7833, 859–860, 13 October 1973.

20. You Can't Live by C Alone

Cheraskin, E., and Ringsdorf, W. M., Jr. (with Brecher, A.) *Psychodietetics.* 1976. New York, Bantam Books. Pp. 155–194. (Originally published by Stein and Day)

——, ——, and Clark, J. W. *Diet and Disease.* 1968. Emmaus, Pennsylvania, Rodale Books. Pp. 65–84.

Conn, R. Too Many Vitamins? (Vitamin C and Iron Absorption). Wichita *Eagle*, Wednesday, 9 July 1980.

Foods High in Sugar and Refined Carbohydrates. Form D2109, 1979. Dietronics, Richardson, Texas.

Harte, R. A., and Chow, B. Dietary Interrelationships. In Wohl, M. G., and Goodheart, R. S., Editors. *Modern Nutrition in Health and Disease.* Third Edition. 1964. Philadelphia, Lea and Febiger. Pp. 534–544.

Jacobson, M. F. *Nutrition Scoreboard: Your Guide to Better Eating.* 1975. New York, Avon Books.

Novey, D. Mixing and Matching Vegetable Proteins. *Nutrition for Optimal Health Association Newsletter* 4:3, Summer 1979.

Sayers, M. H., Lynch, S. R., Charlton, R. W., and Bothwell, T. H. Iron Absorption from Rice Meals Cooked with Fortified Salt Containing Ferrous Sulphate and Ascorbic Acid. *British Journal of Nutrition* 31:3, 367–375, May 1974.

Sayers, M. H., Lynch, S. R., Charlton, R. W., Bothwell, T. H., Walker, R. B., and Mayet, F. The Fortification of Common Salt with Ascorbic Acid and Iron. *British Journal of Haematology* 28:4, 483–495, December 1974.

Sayers, M. H., Lynch, S. R., Jacobs, P., Charlton, R. W., Bothwell, T. H., Walker, R. B., and Mayet, F. The Effects of Ascorbic Acid Supplementation on the Absorption of Iron in Maize, Wheat and Soya. *British Journal of Haematology* 24:2, 209–218, February 1973.

Traub, L. G., and Odland, D. D. *Convenient Food Cost Update*. National Food Review 9, 17–20, Winter 1980.

Index